AGELESS ATHLETE SERIES

CYCLING
Past 50

Joe Friel, MS
Performance Associates Corp.

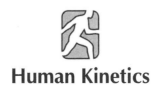

Human Kinetics

Library of Congress Cataloging-in-Publication Data

Friel, Joe.
    Cycling past 50 / Joe Friel.
       p. cm. -- (Ageless athlete series)
    Includes bibliographical references (p.) and index.
    ISBN 0-88011-737-0
    1. Cycling. 2. Cycling--Training. 3. Middle aged persons-
  -Recreation. I. Title. II. Series.
    GV1043.7.F75 1998
    796.6--dc21   97-38749
                                            CIP

ISBN-10: 0-88011-737-0
ISBN-13: 978-0-88011-737-1

Developmental Editor: Kristine Enderle; **Assistant Editor:** Laura Hambly; **Copyeditor:** Denelle Eknes; **Proofreader:** Sarah Wiseman; **Indexer:** Joan Griffitts; **Graphic Designer:** Robert Reuther; **Graphic Artist:** Tara Welsch; **Photo Editor:** Boyd LaFoon; **Cover Designer:** Keith Blomberg; **Photographer (cover):** Beth Schneider; **Photographer (interior):** Tom Roberts (pp. 100, 205); **Illustrators:** Joe Bellis and Paul To; **Printer:** United Graphics

Human Kinetics books are available at special discounts for bulk purchase. Special editions or book excerpts can also be created to specification. For details, contact the Special Sales Manager at Human Kinetics.

Printed in the United States of America   27

The paper in this book is certified under a sustainable forestry program.

Human Kinetics
Web site: http://www.humankinetics.com/

United States: Human Kinetics P.O. Box 5076, Champaign, IL 61825-5076
800-747-4457
e-mail: humank@hkusa.com

Canada: Human Kinetics, 475 Devonshire Road Unit 100, Windsor, ON N8Y 2L5
800-465-7301 (in Canada only)
e-mail: info@hkcanada.com

Europe: Human Kinetics, 107 Bradford Road, Stanningley, Leeds LS28 6 AT, United Kingdom
+44 (0) 113 255 5665
e-mail: hk@hkeurope.com

Australia: Human Kinetics, 57A Price Avenue, Lower Mitcham, South Australia 5062
08 8372 0999
e-mail: info@hkaustralia.com

New Zealand: Human Kinetics. P.O. Box 80, Torrens Park, South Australia 5062
0800 222 062
e-mail: info@hknewzealand.com

E1597

To my wife, Joyce,
for her unwavering love and support

Contents

Acknowledgments

This book would not have happened without the assistance of many people. I'm indebted to Loren Cordain, PhD, of Colorado State University for reviewing the chapter on diet; to sport psychologist Gary Faris for offering suggestions for the mental skills chapter; to Arnie Baker, MD, for arranging contact with the RAAM riders; to Tudor Bompa, PhD, for his insights into the principles of periodization; to Charles Pelkey of VeloNews for the details on Greg LeMond's career; to Gale Bernhardt, my business associate, for reviewing several parts of the work; to Ted Miller and Kristine Enderle of Human Kinetics for their unflappable support and guidance throughout the project; and to my wife, Joyce, for her many hours reading rough drafts and for enduring my endless hours at the computer.

Most of all, I would like to thank the many athletes, now in their 50s, with whom I trained and competed, and who I coached. You taught me well.

Introduction

Do you remember your first bike? Mine was a green Schwinn with white-sidewall tires, a chrome "gas tank," a leather saddle with springs, chrome fenders with mud flaps, a cool chain guard, and multicolored streamers splaying from the white grips. This beauty, a cruiser, was a Christmas present in 1950. Of course, we didn't call it a cruiser back then; it was just a bike.

That bike and I explored and enlarged the unknown world beyond Home Avenue in Greenwood, Indiana, for the better part of 10 years. We went off-road in the woods long before such riding was mainstream, we ran errands to the grocery store, we played for hours on the street in front of my house. After school the green Schwinn was always there eagerly waiting for me.

That Schwinn was my first love affair at age seven. But as young lovers often do, I jilted my Schwinn for a Ford in 1959. Actually, we had been breaking up for a couple of years before as bikes weren't cool at age 14 and 15. I used my green Schwinn less and less until it was finally given to some other kid after Mom got tired of walking around it in the garage.

It wasn't until 1974 that I rediscovered how much fun riding a bike is. For nine years my on-again, off-again infatuation with riding included commuting to work; long, day rides in the mountains; and an occasional camping trip. In 1983 the love affair once again became a passion when I purchased my first real road racing bike.

I soon started racing. That lead to an endless stream of new bike purchases with each one a little higher tech, and more expensive, or meant for a specific purpose. Now I own five bikes—a road bike, a fixed-gear bike, a mountain bike, a get-around-town bike, and a time-trial bike. I've got wheels of every possible type, including standard spokes, bladed spokes, trispokes, composite spokes and rims, disk wheels, 24-inch wheels, and 700-millimeter wheels. My garage is filled with bike tools, repair stands, spare saddles, extra stems and seat posts, and odd parts that are no longer made. It looks like a bike shop, albeit a messy one. I'm a sucker for bikes.

Along the way, I got a masters degree in exercise science, owned a bike shop, and began coaching triathletes, duathletes, road cyclists, and mountain bikers. At first, people came to me for advice on how to improve fitness. Later, I helped riders of all ages and abilities prepare for centuries, tours, and races. My clients gradually became more serious, until today I train mostly elite amateur and professional athletes. I still love riding a bike and helping those who share my passion get more out of the sport.

Your love of cycling is probably much like mine and may have started decades ago with a bicycle love affair that later blossomed into centuries, tours, racing, or fitness riding. Or, maybe you're new to cycling and have purchased this book to find out more about how to prepare your body for better cycling as you grow with the sport.

Whatever your cycling experience, my purpose in writing *Cycling Past 50* is to help you get more from cycling—more health, more fitness, more years, but especially more fun. Fun means different things to different people. For some, it means winning races. For others, fun is participating in group events and riding strongly. Simply learning more about the human body on a bike is fun for many.

My greatest hope is that you'll feel like a kid at play every time you swing your leg over a bike and start pedaling. It's play that keeps you youthful, regardless of how many candles were on your last birthday cake. Whether it's a green Schwinn with white-sidewall tires or a titanium beam bike with composite wheels, a bicycle is sure to reignite a childlike passion for play while keeping you fit forever.

1

Riding Over the Hill

Fifty. The Big Five-O. Did you ever think you'd be that old? Back in the 1960s you were told not to trust anyone over 30. What about 50? Fifty-year-olds were the establishment. Fifty was your parents. Fifty was over the hill and one foot in the grave. People in their 50s were ancient, they were old geezers. They might as well have been from another planet.

Now you're one of them, but you're not alone. Another American joins you at the half-century mark every seven seconds. You and your age cohorts are on the leading edge of the baby boom generation—those 77 million born between 1946 and 1964. One out of three Americans is a boomer. Like a snake swallowing a mouse, this huge bulge of aging boomers is relentlessly moving toward old age. Those born in the late 1940s are on the leading edge of the bulge and are paving the way for the millions to follow. The oldest boomers are also changing the way Americans think about being 50 years old. Sports participation is one agent of that change.

Continued participation in sports is increasingly popular because society's attitudes about the number 50 are changing. The new crop of 50-year-olds are far more likely to stay involved in sport than their predecessors. American society's interest in health, fitness, and athletics is at an all-time high, and that support buoys participation by all ages. Media coverage of masters and seniors competition by athletes who were headliners in previous decades peaks the desire to stay active. The availability of age-group competition in most sports also encourages participation.

Unlike previous generations, which faced economic hardship, most boomers have had the good fortune, and the time, to engage in sports since they were kids. They didn't start as cyclists. They played baseball, football, basketball, volleyball, or soccer. They were wrestlers, gymnasts, runners, swimmers, jumpers, throwers, or climbers. However, later in life boomers found there was something addictive about riding a bike. For some it was the speed. Few self-propelled athletes in other sports go as fast. Others were attracted by cycling's adventurous nature. Covering a ZIP code or two in a day's ride while exploring new terrain is heady stuff. For many others, riding a bike offered the opportunity to remain physical and fit despite a gimpy knee or other injuries that prevented continuing an original sport.

Whatever the reason, cycling has become a passion. It's hard to imagine life without it. Seeing the world from the seat of a bicycle is unlike any other sport experience. Riding is both emotionally and physically rewarding. It's also challenging. The serious cyclist is challenged to maintain, even improve, riding performance despite increasing age.

50 Physiology

There's something about turning 50 that marks a milestone in life. It's more than just having been around for 18,250 days. For most, 50 is the second time in life when they really consider the concept of age and mortality. The first time was at age 40, but that seemed tame by comparison.

At 50, we note the physical changes that have gradually occurred since the 40th birthday, such as needing reading glasses, thinning and graying hair, and wrinkled skin. Individually, these changes don't mean much, but as we do the inevitable accounting at 50, their accumulation can seem overwhelming. Despite joking about these indicators of aging with friends, we take them seriously and investigate other real or imagined changes.

The obvious external changes are omens of what is happening inside, at the cellular level. During the course of a half century of living, the human body experiences relentless change. Science happily describes and measures this metamorphosis.

Agents of Aging

Why do we age? What causes the visible outward and less obvious but more significant inner changes that lead to reduced capacity for work and eventually to death? Those involved in the science of gerontology have attempted to answer these questions for decades. Such study has produced a number of aging theories.

The ticking clock theory proposes that the aging process is programmed into the genes. Throughout life, the theory goes, events are turned on and off by the clock in the cell's nucleus. Puberty and menopause, predictably timed events, are examples of this programming. Lending support to this

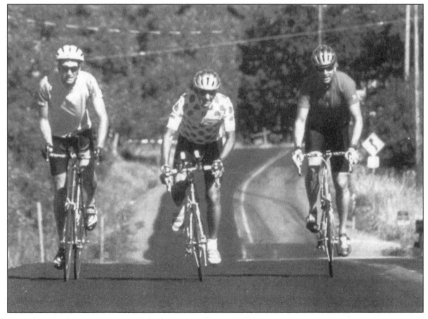

© 1997 Anne Flinn Powell

Cyclists along a country road, climbing over a hill and ready to go!

idea is the research conducted by scientist Leonard Hayflick in 1977. Hayflick showed that a cell can divide a limited number of times and that this is genetically programmed. When cells are no longer able to divide, they die.

Other theories have to do with accumulating damage throughout life. The most popular of these is the free radical theory. Free radicals are products of oxygen metabolism. They are chemical compounds capable of linking with healthy cells, causing oxidative damage similar to metal rusting. According to this theory, the damage accumulates throughout life, killing cells. The proponents of the free radical theory believe that increasing the intake of antioxidants, such as vitamins C and E, reduces free radical damage and thus slows aging.

Blood sugar is sometimes considered a cause of cellular damage and aging. Also called glucose, blood sugar attaches to proteins in abnormal ways, causing cross links and tangles. This leads to many problems associated with aging, such as stiffening tissues, hardening arteries, overly tight ligaments and tendons, cataracts, and atherosclerosis. Because a lifetime of eating a diet high in sweets reduces the body's sensitivity to sugar and its ability to remove and store glucose, the aging process accelerates later in life through accumulated damage.

Slip Sliding Away

Whatever the cause of aging may be, there's little doubt that it eventually produces changes that slow us down. Since the 1930s, scientists have studied the effects of aging on the various systems that comprise human physiology, leading to the following conclusions.

Cardiovascular System

Aerobic capacity is an important aspect of endurance fitness. It's a measure of how much oxygen the body uses to produce energy at a maximal workload. In a lab it's measured as the rider pedals a stationary bike at increasingly higher efforts until continuing is all but impossible. The rider breathes through a tube and oxygen use is measured. The resulting number is called $\dot{V}O_2$max. Elite male cyclists typically have $\dot{V}O_2$max scores in the 70s and 80s (expressed in milli-

liters per kilogram of body weight per minute, or ml/kg/min).
The top women riders score in the mid-60s and 70s.

Starting at about age 20, $\dot{V}O_2$max begins to go down, partly because maximum heart rate, which hits a peak of about 200 beats per minute at age 20, drops by .6 beats per minute each year. This means a drop of 6 beats every decade, so that by age 50 maximum heart rate will have declined by 18 beats per minute. This is true for people who remain moderately active in endurance activity, but the rate is more like one beat per minute per year in couch potatoes, scientists say. Table 1.1 shows the results of age on $\dot{V}O_2$max from one of the earliest studies of this phenomenon. Recent research shows the same relationship.

Not all decline in $\dot{V}O_2$max comes from a reduced heart rate, however. Some loss apparently results from a decrease in the heart's stroke volume, or the amount of blood that it can pump in a single beat. There's about a 3- to 4-percent loss of stroke volume every decade, accompanying the drop in maximum heart rate. The combination of these two means the heart delivers less blood to the working muscles. Less blood means less oxygen is delivered and energy production drops.

Muscular System

Between the ages of 20 and 30, men and women reach their peak strength; then it begins to decline. This is shown in figure

Table 1.1

$\dot{V}O_2$MAX AND AGING

Age (Years)	$\dot{V}O_2$max (ml/kg/min)
25	47.7
35	43.1
45	39.5
52	38.4
63	34.5
75	25.5

Adapted by permission from Robinson, S. 1938. Experimental studies of physical fitness in relation to age. *Arbeitphysiologie* 10: 251-323.

1.1. The primary reason is a loss of muscle mass, about 6 percent per decade after age 30 in sedentary people. Of the two major divisions of muscle type—fast twitch and slow twitch— the fast twitch are lost at a faster rate because individuals are less likely to use them for daily activities. This is a perfect example of the use it or lose it philosophy. When you don't use a muscle for an extended period, the body decides it's more of a burden than a benefit and allows the muscle to wither.

Also lost with aging is muscle elasticity and joint mobility. Failure to regularly use a joint through its full range of movement year after year eventually results in a stiffening of the joint capsule and a loss of muscle, tendon, and ligament function at the extremes of flexion and extension. For the aging weekend warrior or the person returning to riding after several years away from the sport, this can mean an increased risk of injury.

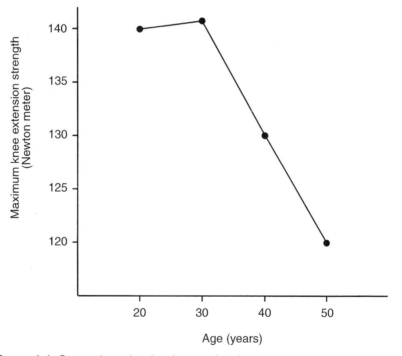

Figure 1.1 Strength and aging in untrained men

Adapted from the *Journal of Neurological Sciences,* 84, J. Lexell et al., What is the cause of the aging atrophy?, 275-294, 1988, with kind permission of Elsevier Science-NL, Sara Burgerhartstraat 25, 1055 KV Amsterdam, The Netherlands.

The good news is that muscles' qualitative parameters remain relatively constant. The muscle of a 50-year-old rider has about the same ability to use oxygen from the blood as the muscle of a 25-year-old pro. The number of capillaries per unit of muscle, and the oxidative enzymes within the muscles necessary to convert oxygen to energy, apparently stay the same.

Pulmonary System

Inhaling brings oxygen-rich air into the lungs, where it enters the blood for eventual distribution to the working muscles. Also in the lungs, carbon dioxide, which is a by-product of metabolism, is released from the blood and returned to the air with each exhale. Maximal expiratory ventilation is a measure of how much air you can breathe in one minute. Aging in sedentary people reduces the elasticity of the lung's tissues, increases resistance to airflow in the airway, stiffens the chest wall, and reduces the strength of breathing muscles. As a result, maximal expiratory ventilation declines with age, starting at about age 20 to 30, and by age 60 is approximately half its peak volume.

Anaerobic System

When riding hard, as in climbing a hill, sprinting, or riding all out, you produce energy anaerobically. The fuel for this energy comes primarily from the breakdown of carbohydrate stored in the muscles and blood. With advancing age, the enzymes necessary to release the energy from carbohydrate decrease, stunting anaerobic potential.

During anaerobic exercise, lactic acid created by the muscles seeps into the blood, from which it must be cleared rapidly or it causes great discomfort and fatigue. It appears that this lactic acid is not carried away as rapidly in older individuals. The bottom line is that hard efforts are increasingly difficult to maintain.

Miscellaneous

In addition to these changes, aging decreases tolerance to heat extremes. The past-50 cyclist sweats less than younger riders in dry, hot conditions. This may be from drier, less oily skin, which swells in such conditions, closing off sweat ducts, raising internal body temperature, and raising the risk of heat injury.

The older person produces more urine, even during exercise, which leads to reduced blood volume. Reduced blood volume means lower capacity for aerobic exercise because less oxygen and fuel can be transported to the working muscles. To compensate for this, heart rate rises rapidly.

Aging seems to weaken the immune system, as the enzymes necessary to maintain healthy function are reduced. So, older riders may be more susceptible to illness and have a harder time fighting it off.

After about age 20, both men and women who remain sedentary gain excess body fat. Even among those who continue to exercise, body fat increases. Figure 1.2 illustrates how body fat changes in relation to age, and figure 1.3 shows how these changes impact $\dot{V}O_2$max. Notice in figure 1.3 that

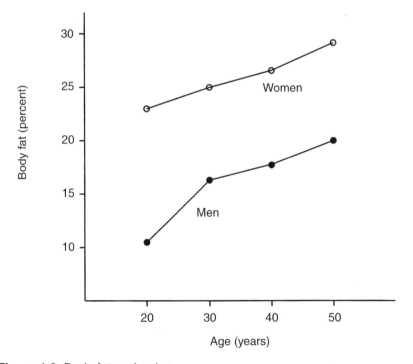

Figure 1.2 Body fat and aging

From Costill, D. 1986. *Inside Running: Basics of Sports Physiology.* New York: McGraw-Hill. Adapted by permission.

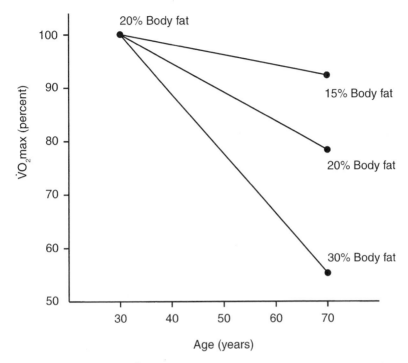

Figure 1.3 Changes in V̇O₂max for different body compositions

when body fat decreases from 20 to 15 percent, V̇O₂max drops little between the ages of 30 and 70. When body fat increases from 20 to 30 percent, V̇O₂max is almost cut in half.

How do the physiological changes described here impact riding a bike? One way of determining that is to look at the age-group records and see what changes take place. Cycling, however, is not an easily measured sport like running, rowing, or swimming, since it is mostly head-to-head competition. Only the individual time trial provides information on aging. Based on male and female records for 40-kilometer races, race times slow at an average rate of 20 seconds per year after age 35, as shown in figure 1.4. So, between ages 40 and 50 you could expect to lose 200 seconds, or about 3 minutes. For a one-hour race, that represents a decline of 5 percent.

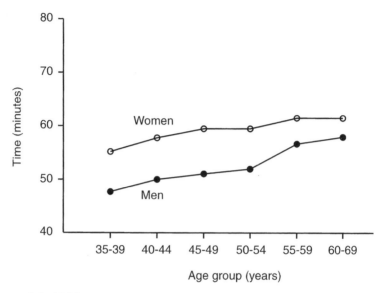

Figure 1.4 1996 age-group records of the United States Cycling Federation 40K time trial

Aging Myth

From all this scientific data, it appears that there is an inevitable decline with aging. Few scientific studies, however, have examined the issue of aging, and most that have were far from perfect. Practically all research studies that looked at aging were cross sectional, meaning they used subjects who were assumed representative of their age groups. For example, a group of 30-year-olds and a group of 50-year-olds were tested for $\dot{V}O_2$max, and the resulting difference was assumed a normal drop due to aging. The same was done on all other aging parameters. It makes sense to conduct a study this way, as the research alternative of following individual people for years, known as longitudinal research, would require decades to gather information.

Cross-sectional studies, however, raise the issue of who the subjects were. What were their lifestyles like? How did they exercise? When a study says they were "trained endurance athletes," which is typical of the language in studies, what does that mean? It's difficult to quantify a subject's degree of training, so most studies use the quantity of training, for example, how often they train and how many weekly miles they cover, to describe the subjects' physical proficiency. Intensity, being a quality measure, is seldom discussed because it's so difficult to quantify, but intensity may be the key to aging.

In fact, it appears that intensity is the most important variable for issues of performance with advancing age. A few examples illustrate this point.

One of the first longitudinal studies was done at Harvard and included a runner named Don Lash. In 1936, at age 24, he held the world record for the two-mile run at 8 minutes, 58 seconds. At that time his $\dot{V}O_2$max was measured at an exceptionally high 81.4 ml/kg/min. After graduating from college, Lash continued to run about 45 minutes daily, but at a greatly reduced pace. In 1961, at age 49, Lash's $\dot{V}O_2$max was measured again, and this time it was 54.4—a drop of about 27 percent in 25 years. That's not too bad considering his contemporaries in the study who also ran in college, but had

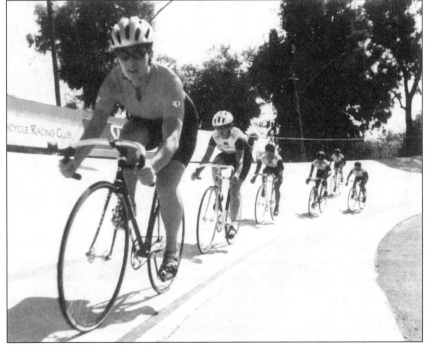

© 1996 Paul Hara

Tara Spangler and the Valley Spokesmen Women's Race Team train at the Hellyer Park Velodrome in San Jose, California.

long since stopped, experienced a 43 percent decline. So, it's apparent that maintaining a moderate volume of exercise keeps some parameters of fitness, such as $\dot{V}O_2$max, fairly constant despite aging. However, it's possible that Lash could have done even better.

Take the example of Hal Higdon, another runner. At age 36, while he was training for the 1968 Olympic Marathon Trials, Higdon's $\dot{V}O_2$max was tested at 67.6 ml/ kg /min by Dr. David Costill at his lab in Dallas. Fourteen years later, at age 50, Higdon's $\dot{V}O_2$max was again tested by Costill and found to have remained high at 63.7. His consistent racing times throughout these years also reflected this excellent maintenance of aerobic function. Higdon was training at age 50 much as he had at age 36, meaning that both his volume and intensity remained high.

Then there's the case of Dr. Costill, himself. In college, in his early 20s, he was a competitive swimmer, yet he accomplished all his personal best times after age 45. At age 22 he swam 1,500 meters in 23 minutes, 31 seconds. After turning 50, he covered the same distance in 19 minutes, 42 seconds. The same goes for his running. His best time for 10 kilometers at age 32 was 43 minutes, 16 seconds, but at age 46 he ran it in 40 minutes, 18 seconds. What happened? After 45, Costill was training at a greater volume and intensity than he had as a young man, and his performances showed it.

Now you could say Higdon and Costill are exceptional cases and unlikely representatives of 50-year-old athletes. Well then, let's take a look at the longitudinal research of Dr. Michael L. Pollock. His 10-year studies attempted to differentiate between fitness losses attributable to aging and those resulting from disuse.

RAAM TOUGH

Too old you say? Big challenges are for kids, you think? How about doing what no one has ever done before? That's the challenge four women in their 50s took on in 1996—the Race Across America as a team. It had never been accomplished, and some thought middle-aged women, especially without experience in ultradistance racing, couldn't do it. They were wrong.

The Race Across America (RAAM) is a brutal, nonstop, coast-to-coast bicycle race from Irvine, California, to Savannah, Georgia—2,904 miles. Begun in the 1980s as an event strictly for solo riders battling climate and sleep deprivation, it has, since 1992, included a team category. Four riders take turns, with each averaging 100 miles a day over mountains and plains, heat and wind, day and night—not your normal tour or race.

The four past-50 women came together when Phyllis Cohen, 53, a comedy writer from Santa Monica, California, sparked the group with a newsletter article. That brought E-mail responses from three eager women—Celeste Callahan, 53, a writer from Denver; Sharon Duncan Koontz, 53, a research analyst from Charlotte, North Carolina; and Jeanette Marsh, 54, an accountant from Starkville, Mississippi. Team W4 included four busy, career-oriented women, two of whom were grandmothers. Two, Celeste and Sharon, were triathletes who had several Ironman Triathlon competitions on their resumes. Before training for RAAM, Phyllis and Jeanette rode for fitness and fun.

On August 4, 1996, they arrived at the RAAM starting line with thousands of miles of hard riding in their legs. Designed by Dr. Arnie Baker, a coach from San Diego, their training was based on 200- to 500-mile weeks of riding 60 to 100 miles a day, weightlifting, cross-training, and mind-numbing indoor rides. The program called for riding twice a day in all kinds of weather and putting in some 200-mile weekends. Maintaining career and family responsibilities was difficult with such a training load. Along the way, there were crashes, dog bites, saddle sores, emotional breakdowns—and even an attack. A passenger in a van hit Jeanette with a two- by four-inch board. It wasn't easy getting to the starting line.

It also wasn't easy getting to the finish line. Riding in two-woman, four- to six-hour rotations, covering about 10 miles per rider at a time, they faced seemingly endless miles of road day after day. Along the way they overcame problems with communications between the four support vehicles, refueling and rest needs, illness, mechanical breakdowns, sunburn, indigestion, flat tires, and organizational issues. But they made it. Seven days, 17 hours, and 30 minutes after starting, Team W4 arrived in Savannah, Georgia, with a rising sun. Their time is now the transcontinental team record for women older than 50.

Would they do it again? Maybe, maybe not. Since RAAM '96, all have returned to normal life, including jobs, grandchildren, hobbies, and, of course, cycling.

In the early 1970s, Dr. Pollock tested 24 men, mostly runners aged 45 to 65. Ten years later they were given the same battery of tests. During the period between the two tests, the men continued to work out, and their training was documented yearly in terms of frequency, intensity, and time. At the time of the second testing in the early 1980s, the subjects were divided into two groups. The competitive group continued to race during the 10 years, and the intensity of their training remained high. After 10 years, their average training pace was within 30 seconds per mile of their original effort. The second group was termed postcompetitive, as they had stopped racing. Their training volume also remained fairly constant, but they ran 90 seconds per mile slower 10 years after the initial exam. Training intensity had dropped considerably for this group.

Table 1.2 summarizes the major differences observed in the two groups as reported in the *Journal of Applied Physiology* in 1987.

Table 1.2

PHYSICAL CHANGES IN COMPETITIVE AND POSTCOMPETITIVE ATHLETES AFTER 10 YEARS

	COMPETITIVE		POSTCOMPETITIVE	
	Test 1	**Test 2**	**Test 1**	**Test 2**
Average age	50.2	60.0	53.9	62.4
Height	5'8.5"	5'8.5"	5'10.25"	5'9.5"
Weight (lb)	148.5	146.7	158.8	155.5
$\dot{V}O_2$max (ml/kg/min)	54.2	53.3	52.5	45.9
Maximum heart rate	177	170	170	163
Body fat (percent)	11.6	13.6	14.3	16.3
Thigh girth	21.3"	21.7"	21.5"	21.3"
Bicep girth	12.3"	12.0"	12.0"	11.9"
Waist girth	31.8"	32.3"	32.4"	33.6"
Resting heart rate	47.6	42.0	50.5	51.9
Systolic blood pressure	117	118	127	138
Diastolic blood pressure	80	79	79	80

From Pollock, M. et al. 1987. Effect of age and training on aerobic capacity and body composition of masters athletes. *Journal of Applied Physiology* 62 (2): 727-728. Adapted by permission.

Both groups did well with their health measures when compared with the average population for the same age groups. Indeed, remaining active is important for staying fit and healthy, as evidenced by the subjects' relatively unchanging weight, percent body fat, and girth measurements. There are, however, several notable differences between the two groups in this study.

Notice, first of all, that the $\dot{V}O_2$max measurements of the competitive group hardly changed. On average, they lost little more than 1 percent of their aerobic capacities in 10 years, while the postcompetitive group saw a 12-percent decline. That's a gigantic difference.

Another measure of aerobic function is resting heart rate. Note that the competitive group's resting heart rate dropped by more than five beats, one good sign of a healthy heart. The resting heart rates of the postcompetitive group stayed much the same.

Percent body fat, and biceps and waist measurements, show that some upper body muscle mass was lost by both groups while they added a little fat around the middle. Notice, however, that the competitive group increased the size of their thighs. This is important as the largest muscles in the body are in the upper leg. It has a major influence on how many calories you burn during the day and the ease with which you do everyday chores, such as carrying groceries up a flight of stairs.

Blood pressure readings remained constant for the competitive group, but the systolic blood pressure of the postcompetitive subjects rose.

Dr. Pollock's study demonstrates that when individuals maintain training intensity, or even increase it as some of the competitive subjects may have done, the scientific measures of fitness are also maintained or even improved. Figure 1.5 shows how these subjects faired in comparison with what we might expect in normal athletic and sedentary populations based on other studies. Notice especially that the competitive group, which aged from 45 to 55 years during the study, beat the odds by improving $\dot{V}O_2$max. In addition, in each competitive subgroup the absolute measures at the end of 10 years, and the rate of change experienced, were superior.

Pollock's study is not an isolated example of the value of intensity when it comes to aging. Other research has found

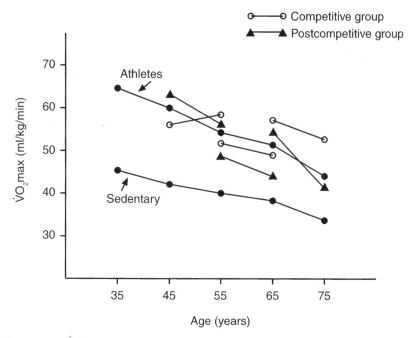

Figure 1.5 $\dot{V}O_2$max of aging athletes

From Pollock, M. et al. 1987. Effect of age and training on aerobic capacity and body composition of masters athletes. *Journal of Applied Physiology* 62 (2): 729. Reprinted by permission.

comparable results. For example, in 1982 Legwold showed that competition-oriented, high-intensity training resulted in only a 2-percent loss of $\dot{V}O_2$max in 10 years for past-50 runners. Those who ran but without the high intensity of the competitive group experienced a startlingly high 13-percent decline in $\dot{V}O_2$max in 10 years.

Bottom Line

The handwriting is on the wall. It appears that much of the slowing that occurs after age 50 is not due to age, but rather to self-imposed limitations. About half the loss is because of inactivity, and perhaps a fourth results from reduced intensity. So, disuse is the greater cause of the commonly accepted performance drop-off that accompanies aging. Advancing years may only account for a quarter of the physiological losses, approximately 2.5 percent in a decade.

Vigorous and frequent riding is what it takes to maintain functional potential, both on the bike and for life in general. Vigorous riding keeps the heart's stroke volume high and the blood vessels clear and elastic. Pushing yourself a bit on the bike will keep the lungs working efficiently. Frequently using muscles near their maximum capacity on the bike and in the weight room will prevent the loss of muscle tissue.

Vigor is the key. Although riding easily is good for slowing the aging process and necessary at regular times for all riders, it is inadequate to keep the loss of function and health that accompanies old age at a minimum. A sensible program that combines high-intensity training, such as hills and intervals, with strengthening, stretching, a sound diet, and adequate recovery is required to counteract the downside of aging and increase the quantity and quality of life.

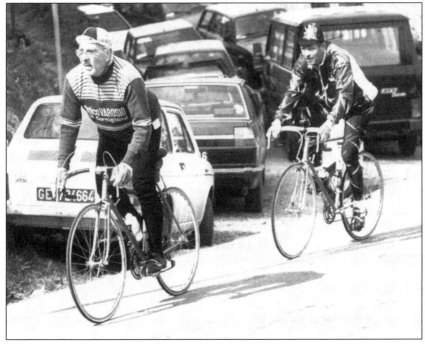

© 1990 Beth Schneider

Cyclists warm up before the 1990 Milano-San Remo race.

Age Not

The decade from age 50 to 60 is the most critical time in life to stay fit and healthy. Here are seven simple rules to help you enjoy riding a bike throughout this decade and for a long time to come. Later chapters of this book describe each rule in greater detail.

- Rule 1. Ride frequently. The most basic element of health and fitness is regular exercise. Don't let your bike collect dust. Try to wear one out every four or five years. The more often you have to replace bikes, the healthier and fitter you will become.

- Rule 2. Rest regularly. Frequent riding demands a balance of regular resting. Keeping a balance between stress and rest is necessary for physical improvement.

- Rule 3. Set challenging goals. Expect nothing but the best from yourself whether on or off the bike.

- Rule 4. Eat like a hunter-gatherer. Get back to eating at Mother Nature's original training table: lots of fresh fruits, vegetables, lean meats, and water.

- Rule 5. Believe in yourself. Remember that you have a lot going for you as a past-50 cyclist, especially the wisdom that comes from experience. See each day as a golden opportunity to grow and gain new experiences.

- Rule 6. Seek the support of others. Surrounding yourself in all walks of life with enthusiastic, knowledgeable, and positive people will keep you joyful and focused.

- Rule 7. Don't slow down. Aging need not be characterized by poor health and rapidly decreasing fitness. Vigor and high energy are strong medicine. Take them regularly.

chapter

2

Born to Ride

For most past-50 cyclists, money isn't the limiter it was when they were younger. The greater challenge is time. Some who retired early have too much and aren't sure how to make the best use of it. For most, it's the opposite; there's never enough time in the day to fit everything in, including time on the bike.

Too Busy to Ride

Let's face it. By the time you've reached 50 or so, you've either made it to the top in your profession, or you aren't going to. Being at the top of your profession has many rewards, but there is a price to pay. For most successful, career-oriented people there is a sad malady called *task creep* in which the hapless sufferers slowly but surely take on more responsibilities than they can complete in the time available. The cure for task creep is delegation, but few use it. Of course, life's chores aren't just work-related; there are also family responsibilities, home maintenance, meal preparation, and community commitments. The combined weight of this burden results in a life spent trying to beat the clock, but the clock always wins.

If you're a victim of task creep, you pine for the time to ride your bike and keep hoping the day will miraculously expand. Somehow, it never does. With judicious daily planning you may have figured out how to make the best use of lunch breaks and weekends to fit in rides. You may even be cutting sleep short to ride your indoor trainer at 5 A.M. If you travel, you may be a master at finding hotels with stationary bikes and squeezing in a few minutes a day. All in all, you may have figured out how to wedge four hours or so of riding into your hectic schedule. How can you best use that time to stay in good enough shape to ride respectably in the tour, century, or race you have planned?

The first thing you must do, if you haven't already, is eliminate all nonbike types of training from your schedule so you can focus your precious training time on the fitness most specific to your event—riding a bike. That means cutting out weightlifting and cross-training. Spend the little time you have firmly affixed to a bike saddle. That will give you the best return on your time invested.

Beyond this obvious change, it is necessary to ride wisely. There's no room for mistakes or wasted saddle time. You must make the best use of every minute. Here are some suggestions for getting the most return from limited time.

It appears from scientific studies that the minimum number of rides in a week should be three. Less than that and aerobic capacity, an important measure of endurance fitness, doesn't improve. The critical frequency, however, seems to be four workouts a week. In fact, one study found that by increasing weekly workouts from three to four, there was nearly a tripling of the average increase in fitness. That's an important lesson to remember when time is short.

Beyond four workouts a week, the improvement rate of aerobic capacity decreases. Note that this is the *rate* of improvement and not the *absolute level* of attainment. In other words, aerobic capacity continues to rise at five, six, or seven weekly workouts, but not as fast as it did when going from three to four rides a week.

Other studies have shown that when initially establishing fitness levels, as just starting to ride a bike, it's best to work out five or six times a week to speed the process. It will take 10 to 12 weeks to get aerobic capacity up to decent levels at this frequency.

How long should a ride last if you have limited time to train? If you use the time judiciously, you can accomplish a lot of fitness in 30 to 45 minutes. That allows time for a 10-minute warm-up, 15 to 30 minutes of focused riding (explained shortly), and 5 minutes to cool down.

Don't forget, however, that cycling is primarily an endurance sport. It doesn't matter how fast you are when redlined and breathing heavy if you don't have the endurance to finish the ride. Somehow, you've got to get in longer rides to build this endurance. Ninety minutes is about the minimum for long rides, and longer is better, depending on the length of the event for which you're training. Early in the year, these should be weekly rides. Once you establish aerobic endurance, you can maintain it with an every-other-week pattern.

The difficulty of the ride is the most critical aspect of training for the rider with limited time. Riding at intensities greater than 90 percent of aerobic capacity, which means just starting to breathe hard, brings substantial increases in fitness. Training at this level is typical of intervals, hill climbing, and sprint workouts. (Chapter 4 describes these and other intense workouts.)

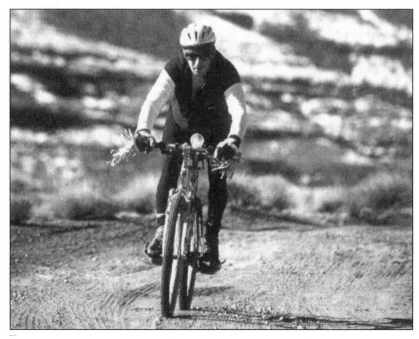

© 1996 Richard Etchberger

Riding off-road keeps you young and spirited. The tassels help too.

It's possible to ride at these high intensities too frequently for too long, causing injury, overtraining, or burnout. Accumulating 30 to 60 minutes a week of riding with the heart rate near or higher than lactate threshold is about all the high-intensity time you need for good fitness.

So, if you ride long once a week, probably on the weekend, and do three high-effort rides during the week, including some with 10 to 20 minutes of high heart rates and heavy breathing, your fitness will stay high or even improve despite limited time. It's probably best to ride intensely only twice a week and make every third week a period of reduced effort to break the routine.

Your Cycling Status

Whether you've got too little time to ride, are just returning to riding, or merely wanting to get more fit for cycling after celebrating your 50th birthday, the journey begins by knowing where you are now. Only then can you make decisions about where you want to go and how to get there. The remainder of this chapter will help you determine your current status, and subsequent chapters will get you started down the road to better fitness.

Red Flags

The first chapter proposed that better cycling fitness, and even improved health, are partially the result of high-effort riding. Some would argue that such physical exertion is risky for people in their 50s. The real issue, however, isn't what's safe for other 50-year-olds to do, but rather what *you* should do.

If you've been riding for several years, especially with regular, high-intensity efforts, there's little reason to believe you can't continue beyond age 50. Then again, our bodies can change as we get older, mostly because of the overindulgence of a comfortable lifestyle. Regardless of your cycling experience, it's best to pause and assess the current status of your health. Even if you are extremely fit, we recommend regular visits to your doctor for physical checkups and perhaps an exercise stress test to get periodic snapshots of your physical well-being, especially the cardiovascular system.

When you're exceptionally fit, it's hard to imagine there could be something wrong with the old body. That's what Jim Fixx, the author of the 1970s best-selling book, *The Complete Book of Running*, believed. At age 36, Fixx took up running—serious running, including 70-mile weeks and numerous marathons. He eventually lost 60 pounds, quit smoking, improved his diet, and lowered the stress in his life. He became fabulously fit. Yet, at age 52, he died while out for a run on a lonely country road in Vermont. Sixteen years of leading an exemplary lifestyle, including lots of aerobic exercise, was not enough to overcome the changes that were occurring in his body.

An autopsy showed that Fixx had probably experienced a heart attack shortly before his tragic Vermont run. It also showed that one of his coronary arteries was nearly 100-percent blocked and another was 80-percent occluded. There were other indicators of his condition. He had an elevated cholesterol count, and his father died at age 43 of a heart attack. The cards were stacked against him.

Heart disease is the leading cause of mortality in the United States, accounting for nearly one-third of all deaths. What are the chances you have hidden heart disease? Knowing your risk level provides a clue as to how cautious you should be with diet, exercise, weight control, and other health factors in your life. There are several determinants of risk. Some are hereditary, others are controllable. Although you can't change heredity, you can modify lifestyle.

We can't emphasize strongly enough the importance of having a physical checkup before beginning a strenuous training program such as those described in this book. If you're new to cycling, or planning to increase your participation, share this with your doctor. Besides checking your heart and confirming your readiness to train, the doctor may look for signs of prostate cancer, a particularly common problem in past-50 men, or, for women, breast cancer.

Finding Your Fitness

Once you have a clear picture of your health, the next step is to establish a fitness-level baseline. By regularly repeating the same test, or better, battery of tests, you can measure your progress and identify fitness areas in need of improvement. There are three aspects of fitness that you may check, either with self-tests or in a laboratory. They are *aerobic efficiency*, *aerobic capacity*, and *power*.

It's critical that the procedures you follow for each test be repeatable, otherwise you won't be certain that the measured changes are a result of improving fitness or a new procedure. This includes the amount of rest in the two days before testing, warm-up, equipment, the course you use as a standard, tire pressure, how long since the last meal, and in some cases, the gears you use. Write all of this down so you can repeat it as closely as possible on retests.

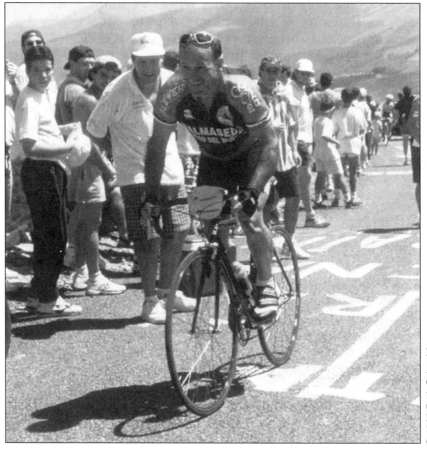

© 1996 Beth Schneider

Fans climb the Port de Larrau before the start of the 1996 Tour de France.

Even with such great care to stabilize the conditions for retests, there will be variables out of your control. For example, tests done outside on the road are subject to wind and temperature changes, and indoor tests are limited by the vagaries of equipment calibration. Even laboratory tests, which are the most likely to be repeatable, can vary considerably. A recent study by Montreal University in Canada found laboratory $\dot{V}O_2$max test results varied by as much as 15 percent from day to day due to calibration errors and faulty equipment. So, even though you keep conditions from one test to the next as constant as possible, there is still room for error. This means that the tests aren't perfect measures of your fitness, but they can be helpful in determining progress.

Aerobic Efficiency Tests

The purpose of the aerobic efficiency tests is to determine whether you're using oxygen and energy economically. As your body becomes more efficient, you require less energy for the same output, or to look at it another way, more output is possible for the same energy input. You can measure input using heart rate and measure output by speed or power. Here are two tests based on this principle that you can do either indoors or on the road.

Aerobic Time Trial. Carefully measure off a three-mile course on a flat section of road that has no stop streets and light traffic. To allow for wind changes, make it 1.5 miles out and back. Warm up 10 to 20 minutes, slowly bringing heart rate up to a predetermined level in the range of 80 to 85 percent of maximum. If you don't know your maximum heart rate, choose one that is moderately difficult to maintain for a long time. Following the warm-up, without stopping or allowing the heart rate to go down, ride the course, carefully watching your heart rate monitor so you stay within the range of one beat higher or lower than the test heart rate. This will be difficult to do at first, but with periodic retesting, you'll get better at it. Keep the gear the same throughout the test. Record your time for the course along with the test heart rate and gear. Improvements in aerobic efficiency will be accompanied by faster times for the course.

You can do the same test on an indoor trainer if you have a rear-wheel sensor for your handlebar computer or equipment such as a RacerMate CompuTrainer or Cycle Ops Electronic Trainer. The CompuTrainer and Electronic Trainer should be calibrated. Standard indoor trainers provide questionable results because they can't be calibrated.

Ramp Test. Another way of determining aerobic efficiency is to do the ramp test on a stationary bike, CompuTrainer, or Electronic Trainer. Or, if your handlebar computer has a rear-wheel speed sensor, you can use a standard indoor trainer. The test involves increasing intensity for four stages, then stopping for one minute. Start at a standard low output such as 50 watts or 12 miles per hour. Every three minutes increase the work output by about 50 watts or 3 miles per hour. Complete four such nonstop stages, for example, 50, 100, 150, and 200 watts. Use the same gear throughout the test. Record heart rate at the end of each stage. After the fourth stage, stop pedaling and record heart rate one minute later. You will now have five heart rates recorded. Add these together for a ramp test score. Improvements in aerobic efficiency will mean a drop in your score. Be sure to write down the wattage or speed levels you used, along with the gear.

Aerobic Capacity Tests

Aerobic capacity is a measure of how much oxygen your working muscles are capable of using. Because oxygen usage is related to energy production, aerobic capacity is a good measure of endurance fitness. The tests for measuring this are the most stressful because they push you to the limit. For this reason, it's a good idea to discuss this test with your physician before completing it. Or, better yet, have the test done in a laboratory.

Time Trial. Choose a day when the wind is calm and the temperature is not high. Don't eat for two hours before, and drink nothing other than water. Warm up 10 to 20 minutes. Then on a flat, three-mile course such as the one used for the aerobic time trial, time yourself while riding as fast as you can. Gear selection is optional, and you can shift at any time during the test. Your time for the test is an indirect measure of your aerobic capacity.

VO_2max Test. Laboratory testing for aerobic capacity, also called $\dot{V}O_2max$, is possible and likely to be more accurate than

the time-trial method. The downside, however, is cost. Expect to pay $150 or more for such a test in a medical clinic. If you have a university nearby, check with the exercise physiology department to see if they are looking for subjects for studies involving $\dot{V}O_2$max testing. Chances are slim, but it's worth a try. Be sure to get tested on a bicycle ergometer and not a treadmill, as $\dot{V}O_2$max is specific to the activity. There is little relationship between running and cycling aerobic capacities.

Of course, knowing the result of one test is interesting information, but tells you nothing about changes in fitness, so regular testing is necessary. For this reason, most riders simply use the time-trial method.

Should you decide to use a clinic for the test, other services are often offered as part of an assessment package. This may include diet analysis and body composition measurement, for example.

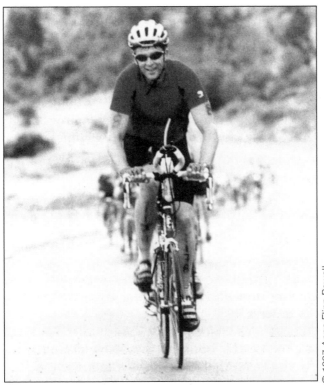

© 1997 Anne Flinn Powell

Over the hill and ahead of the pack, this triathlete is moving!

Power Tests

There's a close relationship between how much power you can generate on a bike and how strong a rider you are. Power is necessary for sprinting and going over short, steep hills. Self-measurement of maximum power requires an assistant or two because you must be totally focused on your effort while testing.

Hill Sprint. Find a short, steep hill of about 6- to 8-percent grade. The hill approaching a highway overpass is about right. Mark off a section of about 50 yards starting from the bottom of the hill. You'll need two assistants, one at the start of the 50-yard course and the second at the finish mark with a stopwatch. After warming up for 10 to 20 minutes, approach the hill at a standard speed of about 18 miles per hour. As you hit the start line your first assistant's hand drops, signaling the second assistant to start a stopwatch. Go as hard as you can up the hill. As you cross the finish mark, the second assistant stops the watch. Your time is an indicator of power. You may want to make three or four attempts in one testing session.

Wingate Test. Some human performance labs, such as at universities and clinics, are equipped to test power using a special procedure called a Wingate Test. Just as with $\dot{V}O_2max$ tests done in a lab, you must repeat the test frequently to check progress, and the expense may soon become an issue.

Indoor Trainer Testing. If you own a CompuTrainer or Electronic Trainer, you can test for power in a more controlled setting than out on the road. The materials that come with these trainers offer instructions for power testing.

Now What?

Repeat tests every six to eight weeks to allow time for measurable change. Don't expect big improvements, especially if you're an experienced rider. A 2- or 3-percent change in two months is quite a bit.

If the results of a test indicate that you're not improving or even going backward, consider first how close the test conditions were to the one you're comparing it with. Also, consider your self-perceptions of fitness in this area. Sometimes you may feel as if you've improved, yet the test says otherwise. Be reluctant to make changes in your training unless you're confident the test is right.

The changes you make depend on the type of test. Poor aerobic efficiency usually improves simply by getting more time in the saddle. Another way to improve it is to ride frequently at the effort levels of the test. Of course, it's important that the test efforts reflect the efforts of the event for which you're training.

You can improve aerobic capacity by doing high-intensity workouts, such as intervals and hilly rides. The heart rates for these workouts should fall in the range of 85 to 95 percent of maximum heart rate. These workouts are described in greater detail in chapter 4.

If you determine that power needs improvement, two or three weekly workouts devoted to increasing strength and quickly turning the cranks will soon remedy this. Leg speed workouts are explained in chapter 4 and weight training is described in chapter 8.

chapter

3

Basic Training

You've probably been riding a bike for a long time and have learned a lot about improving fitness. Experience is a great teacher. In fact, this chapter's discussion of some basic aspects of training for cycling may be old hat—stuff that you learned a long time ago and still use, but never thought about. Then again, there may be something here you've missed. For example, do you understand the ways you can vary on-bike training to change the difficulty level? Have you figured out how you can bring fitness to a peak at the right times in the year? Do you know how to use lactate threshold heart rate to get the optimum benefit from your riding time? These are a few topics explored in this chapter.

The greater the benefits you hope to get from riding a bike, the more you need to know. This chapter introduces several concepts, from experience and from science, that will make you a more knowledgeable rider. This assumes, of course, that you will plan your training rather than just rolling out of the driveway and seeing what happens down the road. Smart planning will make you better on the bike, no matter what your goals are.

Cardinal Rules of Training

Since 1971, I've trained and coached athletes in a variety of sports with abilities ranging from beginner to professional. Some became national- and world-class competitors; others achieved less impressive, but no less important, personal goals. All improved their physical abilities in some way.

I don't know who learned more—me or them. My lessons came from observing how small changes in training brought big results. Some riders obviously had a lot of potential when they came to me. They were highly motivated and did challenging workouts, but for some reason they weren't getting all they could from training. At first this was perplexing. How could athletes with such great potential achieve so little? After years of reviewing hundreds of training logs, I began to see patterns and understand why a person with latent ability was not coming close to attaining it. He or she was breaking one of what I call the Cardinal Rules of Training.

No matter what you want from riding, there are three rules you must obey. Breaking any of these means, at best, limited improvement, and, at worst, overtraining and loss of fitness. The Cardinal Rules of Training are as follows:

- Rule 1. Ride consistently.
- Rule 2. Ride moderately.
- Rule 3. Rest frequently.

These may seem overly simple. Sometimes, however, the most important things in life are the simplest. Such is the case with training.

Rule 1 is based on the premise that nothing does more to limit or reduce fitness than missed rides. The human body thrives on regular patterns of living. When cycling routinely and uniformly progressing for weeks, months, and years, fitness steadily improves. Interruptions from injury, burnout, illness, and overtraining cause setbacks. Each setback means a substantial loss of cycling fitness and time reestablishing a level previously attained. Inconsistent riding is like pushing a boulder up a hill only to see it roll back down before reaching the top—frustrating.

Riders who violate the first rule of training are usually frustrated. The solution to their problem is simple: Train consistently. "Okay," they say, "but how do I do that?" Good question, and that leads to the other Cardinal Rules. The second Rule, ride moderately, is the first step in becoming more consistent. This one usually scares highly motivated, hard-charging cyclists. They can see themselves noodling around the block in slow motion and not even working up a sweat. However, that's not what moderate means.

Moderate riding is that level of training to which your body is already adapted, plus about 10 percent. For example, if the longest recent ride is 40 miles, then a reasonable increase is to 45 miles next week. That's moderate. A 60-mile ride would not be moderate and could lead to something bad, such as an injury or overtraining that forces several days off the bike and a lapse in consistency. Another moderate change is steadily progressing from riding flat terrain to rolling hills, to riding longer hills, to riding steep and long hills. Going from riding on the flats to steep, long hills is not moderate.

Consistent riding also requires frequent resting. That means planning rest at the right times, such as after challenging rides or hard weeks. Chapter 7 discusses this misunderstood

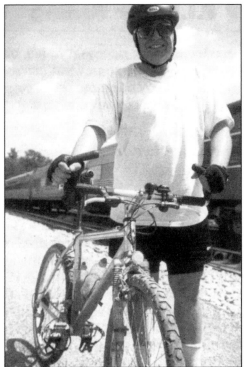

Try a rail to trail line. Heritage Rail Trail, York County, Pennsylvania.

concept in greater detail. Rest taken in adequate doses and at appropriate times produces consistent training and increased fitness.

Even though the Cardinal Rules of Training are basic, if you follow them, fitness will improve regardless of what else you do on the bike. They are deceptively simple to read about; incorporating them into training is a different matter. At first, it may be difficult to ride moderately and rest frequently. Keep working at it. Old habits are hard to break. When you initially train this way, it's better to err on the side of being conservative with moderation and rest if you're a rider who has frequent breakdowns and missed workouts. With experience you'll become better at determining what is right for you.

Although what we have discussed so far came strictly from experience, the following basic components of training come mostly from science.

F.I.T. for Riding

Even though moderation is necessary, it's obvious that a portion of your riding must be somewhat stressful to cause a positive change in fitness. Moderate stress comes from carefully manipulating three workout variables:

- Frequency—how often to ride
- Intensity—how hard to ride
- Time—how long to ride

Frequency

The first question to ask at the start of a week is, "How often should I ride?" Training to race, for example, in the United States Cycling Federation's national age-group championship, requires a different response to this question than if the goal is general health and fitness. The higher the goal for ultimate performance, the more often you need to ride.

Potential is an elusive concept: an ability that is possible but not yet realized. None of us ever knows how close we are to our potential. We do know, however, that getting there demands many sacrifices, one of which involves being on a bike several times a week instead of sitting in front of a TV nibbling on potato chips. When it comes to frequency, there are suggested minimums and maximums, depending on goals. If your reasons for riding are strictly health and basic fitness, the minimum number of rides each week is three. This assumes you ride only and don't cross train. Because training in other aerobic sports has a cardiovascular benefit, you could get away with riding less frequently and still improve the most basic elements of health and fitness.

Other than achieving high levels of fitness, another frequency issue is how to get in shape the fastest. When first starting to train on a bike, five or six rides each week will cause the most rapid change in fitness. Scientific research shows an increase in aerobic capacity, one measure of fitness, of about 43 percent for novices training this frequently. Three to four rides each week bring a 20- to 25-percent improvement.

If you already have a high aerobic capacity from many weeks of consistent training, all you need to maintain it is four rides a week. High-performance racers, however, usually ride five to seven times a week.

Intensity

Regardless of training frequency and time, the single most critical training variable is how hard and fast you ride. There are several ways of measuring intensity. The one you're most likely to have available is heart rate. The greatest changes in aerobic capacity come from training at high heart rates, in excess of 90 percent of maximum. Although the highly motivated athlete often seeks such benefits, frequent training over 90 percent of maximum heart rate obviously violates the Cardinal Rule of moderation and will eventually lead to inconsistency and loss of fitness.

The key to cycling intensity is knowing when to ride at higher heart rates and when to slow down. So, 90 percent plus is the high side, but what about the low end? Riding less than 50 percent of maximum heart rate has little or no impact on aerobic fitness. Such low-effort riding is of little physiological value except, perhaps, for recovery.

Getting intensity right is the trickiest aspect of training. Later, this chapter will teach you how to use a heart rate monitor, and chapters 5 and 6 will pull all pieces of the training puzzle together with suggested routines based on riding goals.

Time

The duration of your rides is the second most effective variable in improving fitness. In fact, there's good reason to believe that longer, slower workouts are equivalent to shorter, faster training sessions in improving aerobic capacity. Because lower intensity workouts are easier on the body, most athletes and coaches recommend building a base of endurance with long, steady rides before starting to do high-intensity workouts, such as intervals, later in the training year.

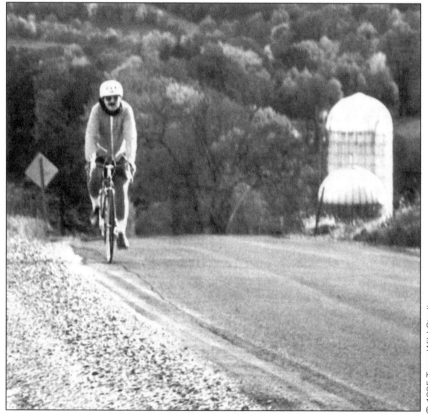

© 1995 Terry Wild Studio

As part of your basic training, do some long rides.

The length of your rides depends on what you're used to. In your first five years of cycling, you should be able to increase riding mileage or time by about 10 percent over the previous year's volume. However, if you've ridden for several years, there's a limit to how many miles you need to improve. Through experience, you may have already discovered that limit—due primarily to an inability to recover and go again.

Periodization

The product of frequency, intensity, and time is called workload. It can be expressed mathematically as the following:

$$\text{Frequency} \times \text{intensity} \times \text{time} = \text{workload}$$

You can change the workload of cycling by increasing any of the three variables and keeping the other two constant. Some coaches and athletes regularly change the components of workload every few weeks to reach a physical peak at certain times of the year. This way of training is known as *periodization* and was the brainchild of sports scientists in the Eastern Block countries of the 1960s.

Today, most serious bike racers subscribe to the idea of periodization, but even if you're not keen on competition, the principles of periodization can help you become a better rider. The three commonly accepted periodization principles basic to endurance training are predictability, pyramiding, and planned rest.

Predictability

Planning to reach a fitness peak at predetermined times of the year is central to periodization. These peak periods may last up to six weeks each. You can achieve two or three such peaks a year by repeating training periods that manipulate and cycle the workload variables of frequency, intensity, and time.

Figure 3.1 illustrates the interplay of intensity and time for a hypothetical rider to create two peaks of fitness within one year. The periodization plan shown here is simple: annual training plans are often created with three peaks and greater variance of intensity and time.

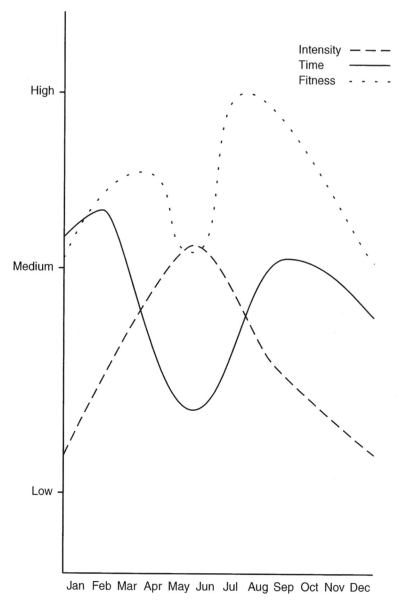

Figure 3.1 Periodization plan to produce two fitness peaks by varying workout intensity and time

Pyramiding

Periodization involves training in multiweek periods to develop the most basic elements of fitness first, then building the more refined fitness components later. Generally, three to six weeks make up one training period. You maintain aspects of fitness improved in previous periods as you develop new ones. For example, early in the year, you could build endurance by gradually increasing the time of workouts as intensity stays low to moderate. In a later period, you could improve speed and power with greater intensity in training while maintaining endurance with less frequent, long rides. Figure 3.2 shows

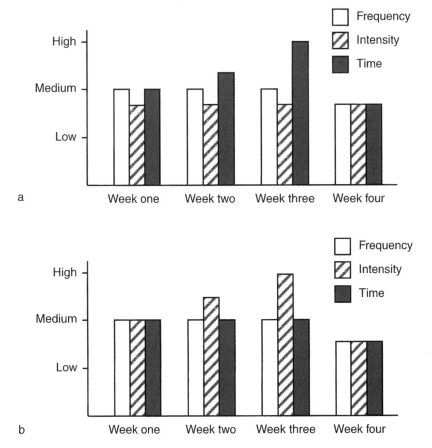

Figure 3.2 Four-week period emphasizing (a) endurance and (b) intensity

how you can vary frequency, intensity, and time to emphasize specific aspects of cycling fitness within a four-week period. Typically, each training period becomes more difficult than the previous as the cyclist builds to a peak.

Planned Rest

Periodization emphasizes the role of frequent periods of rest and recovery for the body to absorb the training of the previous period before embarking on a new, and more challenging, period of riding. In the same way, you can build R and R into the annual calendar. Resting at the right times and in the appropriate ways is critical for the past-50 cyclist.

Real World Periodization

Periodization is well suited for experienced cyclists. First-year riders should vary only frequency and time, and keep intensity low to moderate. After a year or two of building bike endurance, leg strength, and cycling-related skills, you can initiate periodization by gradually increasing the intensity of training.

Experienced cyclists, in the early periods of a training year, increase the frequency and time, keeping intensity on the low side. This improves cardiorespiratory and aerobic endurance in the safest way. Once endurance is high, cyclists reduce training time and increase intensity to produce an even higher fitness level. It generally takes 8 to 12 weeks to develop endurance but only 4 to 8 weeks to see significant improvements in fitness with increased intensity. Once fitness is high, the serious racer further decreases riding time while increasing intensity to bring fitness to a very high peak before important races. Figure 3.3 illustrates the six annual periods and how they vary the workload. Chapter 6 describes periodization plans for experienced racers.

Even if racing is not your focus, the peaking process is beneficial for preparing for any event that will stretch your current fitness level, such as a tour or century. Such events demand a great deal of aerobic endurance, strength for the hills, and muscular endurance for the many miles ahead. Chapter 5 presents periodization plans for these events.

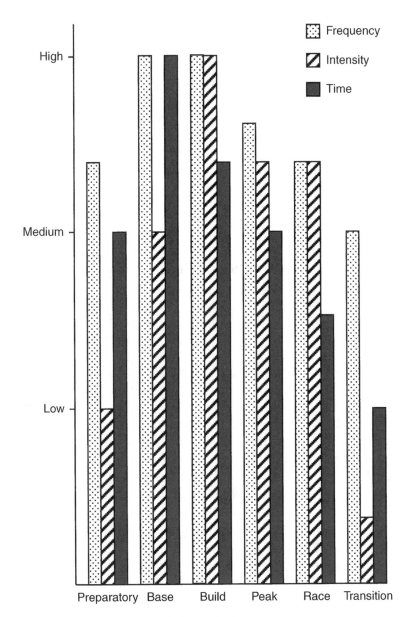

Figure 3.3 Workload changes by period

Principles of Training

The purpose of training is to improve some aspect of cycling performance, whether it is endurance, strength, or speed. Each component requires training in exacting ways to create new levels of fitness. Although it's possible to do this from training by the seat of your pants, planned training is likely to bring higher fitness levels that better match your needs with less wasted time and effort. The following training principles will guide your planning.

Overload and Adaptation

There's an old saying that goes, "What doesn't kill you, makes you stronger." The point is that when physically stressed in some way, the human body adapts and grows more resilient. When talking about bike training, this increased stress is called overload and could come in the form of a longer-than-normal ride, a hard hill workout, or riding more frequently.

Stress is only half of the fitness equation, however, with the other half being rest. It's during rest that adaptation and growth take place at the cellular level, a slow process for those over 50. In the recovery time following a stressful workout, for example, a long ride on a hilly course, hundreds of small changes occur, such as an increase in the enzymes that help metabolize fat and the growth of muscle cells. Without rest there would be no improvement. In fact, without rest, you could count on losing fitness following tough rides.

Figure 3.4 illustrates how you grow stronger as a result of applying a new overload in the form of a challenging ride at Time 0, then allowing a period of rest. Note that between Time 0 and Time 1 there is a loss of fitness accompanied by fatigue. At Time 1, fatigue diminishes as the adaptation process begins, eventually resulting in greater cycling fitness, known as overcompensation, by Time 3. Time 3 is the appropriate time to apply a new overload, causing the pattern to repeat at a higher level than before.

The problems come when new overloads in the form of stressful rides are applied at the wrong times, either too soon (Time 1 or Time 2) or too late (Time 4 or Time 5). The

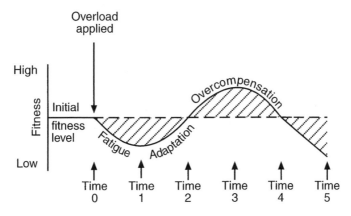

Figure 3.4 Overcompensation from overload and rest

reapplication of a challenging ride, either too early or too late, results in a further loss of fitness. Of these two timing mistakes, the greater error comes from going hard again too soon. This is the more common mistake highly motivated cyclists make, which can lead to overtraining if it's frequently repeated.

Look again at figure 3.1. Notice that both fitness peaks occur in the troughs when time and intensity are moderate. These periods of relative rest allow the body to adapt and grow stronger. Overcompensation results from rest both weekly and seasonally.

Individualization

After learning about the timing of strenuous rides, especially as shown in figure 3.4, the question you must have is, "When is Time 3?" The best time to apply the second overload, as with most questions about training, is an individual matter. It depends on how great the overload was that initiated the fatigue at Time 0, what your riding was like in the days and weeks leading up to that point, how quickly your body recovers, what recovery techniques you use, and what kind of riding you did between Time 0 and Time 2. In addition, there are a myriad of off-the-bike stresses that could affect the timing of the next overload, such as working in the yard, overtime at work, financial worries, or relationship problems, to name a

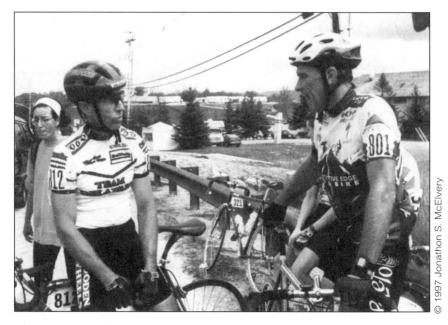

Skip Cutting and Clive Woakes discuss the 1997 Killington Stage Race 50+.

few possibilities. The list of activities that could delay adaptation is endless.

Furthermore, some cyclists are fast responders and others are slow responders. Fast responders need only a short time to adapt, but slow responders need longer. What this means is that if you and a friend of nearly equal ability do a hard ride together, chances are you won't both be 100-percent ready for the next stressful ride at the same time, even if everything else in your lives was the same. Response time slows with aging.

Some generalization about recovery is possible, however. For most past-50 cyclists, the time to do another challenging ride falls between 48 and 72 hours after the first, considering the variables mentioned, especially how difficult the original workout was at Time 0. Chapter 7 will discuss this issue in greater detail.

Training for cycling is an individual matter, and each of us is an experiment with one subject. Doing what another person does, no matter how strong a rider he or she is, doesn't mean that you'll achieve the same level of performance. You must listen to your body.

Specificity

Do you want to ride a long distance, such as a century? Is completing a triathlon your goal? How about traveling across the country—is that your reason for riding? Is basic fitness your objective?

Answering such questions is necessary to plan training. Not having a clear notion of what you want from cycling is a sure way to achieve nothing worth having. Training without a fitness destination in mind is like getting in your car and driving without a clear idea of where you want to go. You will certainly wind up somewhere, but perhaps in a place you don't care to be.

Building greater cycling fitness, regardless of your ultimate use of that fitness, requires a destination and a map, or training plan, for getting there. Knowing what you want makes it easy to determine how to train, because training will reflect your ultimate application. For example, a cyclist aiming for road racing knows it will be necessary to ride three hours nonstop in the race and includes several rides of at least that duration. He or she also knows there will be hills on the course, so rides on hilly terrain. The race may come down to a sprint for the finish line, so training will involve some sprinting.

The idea is that bike workouts must closely match the workload of the event you're training for. This is the principle of specificity.

In the previous road race example, the cyclist knows there won't be any running. Does this mean he or she should never run? There is a time when nonspecific training is beneficial and a time when it is less so. The closer you get to the goal event, the more specific your training must become. Figure 3.5 illustrates this principle. To answer the question about running, figure 3.5 shows that it is best done in the early stages of fitness building, for example, in November and December, and less beneficial in the later stages, such as March and April.

Other examples of nonspecific training for a bike racer are skiing, weightlifting, swimming, hiking, and aerobics classes.

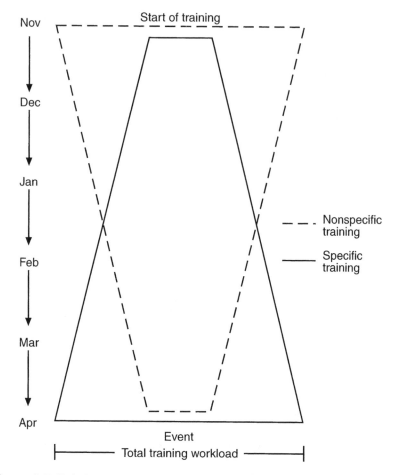

Figure 3.5 Relative volumes of specific and nonspecific training activities during five months of preparation for an event

For a fitness cross-trainer who uses the bike as only one mode of exercise, the term specific is almost meaningless; each activity is appropriate for such a user at any time of the year.

The Heart of Training

Earlier, this chapter discussed intensity and explained how it is the most critical element of training for the experienced cyclist. Knowing how intense a workout is means monitoring some physiological system while riding. There are several possibilities that are closely observed in laboratory stress tests, such as blood lactate measurement and exhaled gases, but when it comes to training in the real world, the best indicator for most riders is heart rate. The remainder of this chapter will teach you how to use a heart rate monitor to train at the appropriate intensity for the benefits you're seeking and how to determine cycling progress using heart rate.

Evolution of Intensity

It is possible to train without a heart rate monitor or any technical method of determining intensity. In fact, you probably rode this way for years with great success, using one or a combination of three methods. The first method used descriptive words such as hard, moderate, or easy. You simply evaluated how you felt while riding, so comparisons with other riders or previous rides were difficult, if not impossible. Another method may have been based on riding at a given pace using a speedometer. This was useful only if the conditions, such as wind and hills, remained constant. Usually they didn't, so a third method became popular with some, called rating of perceived exertion, or RPE. Using this system, a rider would assign an exertion rating to the current effort of the ride, using a scale from 6 to 20 with 6 representing rest and 20 maximal exertion. The range of 6 to 20 was originally selected by scientists because with younger athletes in their 20s, the exertion rating could be multiplied by 10 to estimate heart rate. So, if a young cyclist said he was riding at an RPE of 15, that would predict a heart rate of 150. This system made training a bit more scientific, but relied heavily on the rider's subjective ratings, which were suspect when the excitement of competition was high or motivation varied.

The coming of the heart rate monitor in the early 1980s changed all this. The change didn't come overnight, however, as the devices didn't fully catch on until the early 1990s. It also took a while for cyclists to learn how to use them. At first, heart rate monitors were merely gee whiz toys—fun to play with, but not meaningful. Now that has changed. Heart rate monitoring has become quite sophisticated.

What Heart Rate Indicates

When at rest, heart rate is low. In fact, resting heart rate is one measure of fitness progress and can sometimes suggest where your body is on the overcompensation curve (see figure 3.4). The morning after a challenging ride (Time 1), resting heart rate counted on waking will frequently be up a few beats per minute from your norm. This indicates the increased fatigue discussed earlier. A day or two later, it may drop to normal or even lower than normal on waking, telling you that the time is right for another challenging ride. Unfortunately, resting heart rate is not a foolproof method, so other physical and mental factors need consideration before deciding to train hard again. Chapter 7 describes other methods.

During a ride, heart rate rises at a steady rate as the perceived intensity increases. The reason for this rise is that the heart is trying to keep up with the muscles' demand for fuel and oxygen and maintain body temperature as the working muscles give off heat. The obvious condition you're aware of when working harder is an increase in the breathing rate and depth. The reason you're breathing harder is to get more oxygen to the muscles and eliminate the carbon dioxide the muscles give off as lactic acid, which is converted to lactate in the blood. Lactate production is central not only to understanding how to use a heart rate monitor, but also to optimal training.

CARDIAC DRIFT—WHAT'S UP?

You may have noticed while wearing a heart rate monitor during rides that the beats per minute rise as the workout progresses, even though the speed and effort remain about the same. What's going on here? Is there something wrong with the monitor, or—heaven forbid!—with your heart?

Actually, it's neither. It's just that heart rate is affected by several common endurance factors.

What you're observing is called cardiac drift, and although it is normal for everyone, it has a less deleterious effect on the well prepared. For the unprepared, heart rate can drift up as much as 20 beats, given the right circumstances. There are several causes of this upward trend of the ticker during a ride, including muscular fatigue, heat and humidity, dehydration, and even psychological stress.

Muscular fatigue is a demon lurking around the corner, ready to spring on the next poorly trained rider to come along. When muscular fatigue pounces, the slow twitch muscles, which carry most of the cycling load, are no longer able to contract forcefully enough to move the bike at the desired speed. To compensate for this potential loss of power, the central nervous system recruits other muscles to help. These other muscles are more than likely fast twitch muscles, which produce lactic acid and aren't as well-trained for endurance. The need to remove lactic acid and a resulting less economical pedaling technique cause heart rate to rise.

To cool off in hot and humid conditions, the body shunts blood to the skin, leaving less available for the working muscles. Now with two demands facing it, blood for cooling and for the working muscles, the heart has to pump faster to keep up. Acclimating to heat and humidity considerably reduces the upward drift.

Heat and humidity can also lead to dehydration, another cause of cardiac drift, although low body fluid levels can occur in cold or dry conditions, also. When dehydrated, blood plasma volume is reduced, lowering blood pressure. To maintain blood pressure for working muscles, the heart speeds up to match output to demand. As little as a 2-percent drop in body fluid levels, for example, a 3-pound loss of fluid for a 150-pound rider, can cause cardiac drift. At 4 or 5 percent, an athlete may be forced to stop altogether. Drinking fluids before and every 10 to 15 minutes during a ride helps to prevent this problem.

Another cause of drift is psychological stresses, such as tension, irritability, and anxiety. A close miss by a car, being chased by a dog, or the excitement of a race can all elicit higher heart rates.

Although heart rate is not a perfect indicator of intensity, due to cardiac drift, it is the best option we currently have available.

Lactate Threshold

Your muscles are always creating lactic acid; even while reading this book a small amount is produced. Lactic acid doesn't stay in the muscle cells but seeps out into the bloodstream. When it does, its chemical property changes somewhat, and it is then called lactate. At low levels, as in slow riding, the body easily removes the lactate, shuttling some of it to the liver where it's converted into glycogen for fuel for the muscles in a truly efficient process. As the speed and intensity of the ride increase, lactate production also rises. Lactate levels eventually reach the point at which more is in the blood than the body can quickly remove, so it begins to accumulate. The point at which accumulation starts is called the lactate threshold. You may also see it referred to as anaerobic threshold. At the lactate threshold (LT), lactate starts building up in the blood and you are operating in an anaerobic state, one in which you're more dependent on carbohydrate-based fuels than on fats. What you experience at LT is deep breathing and a slight burning sensation in the working muscles, which on the bike is primarily the quadriceps of the upper thigh.

Your heart rate at LT is an excellent indicator of your body's workload, and you can effectively base training zones on it. The difficult part is determining LT heart rate (LTHR), but once you know it, by simply multiplying a few times, you have heart rate training zones that are associated with specific cycling benefits. No more talking about hard, moderate, and easy rides or ratings of perceived exertion. A quick check of the wrist monitor tells where you are.

There are several ways to estimate LTHR. The easiest, but most expensive, is to have it done in a laboratory setting such as a hospital, medical clinic, or university. The technician will generally measure heart rate and compare it with another known factor such as blood lactate or expired gasses. Expect to pay $150 or more for such a test.

Another way to find LTHR is to perform a self-test using a heart rate monitor and the rating of perceived exertion discussed earlier while riding a stationary bike or your bike mounted on an indoor trainer. The device you use must be capable of accurately indicating some measure of work output, such as miles per hour or watts. Besides this, all you need is a heart rate monitor and an assistant to record the data. See Lactate Threshold Heart Rate Test for the details.

LACTATE THRESHOLD HEART RATE TEST ON TRAINER

You will need an assistant; a bike with a rear-wheel computer pickup; and a magnetic, fluid, or wind load trainer with a high load potential. You may use a stationary bike with speedometer, CompuTrainer, or Cateye CS-1000 Cyclosimulator. Warm up for

10 minutes, then follow these steps:

1. Start at 15 miles per hour. Every minute, increase speed by one mile per hour by pedaling faster or by shifting. Do not stand during the test.
2. At the end of each minute the assistant records your heart rate and rating of perceived exertion (RPE) based on the following scale. Place this scale where you can see it while riding.

Table 3.1

RPE SCALE

6	
7	Very, very light
8	
9	Very light
10	
11	Fairly light
12	
13	Somewhat hard
14	
15	Hard
16	
17	Very hard
18	
19	Very, very hard
20	Maximum

3. Continue increasing speed and recording data in this way until you can no longer maintain speed.
4. Your assistant should listen closely to your breathing to detect when it becomes labored and place a VT (ventilatory threshold) on the data sheet next to the proper stage when this occurs.
5. The data collected should look something like table 3.2.
6. Compare VT heart rate with an exertion rating of 15 to 17 to determine LTHR. If VT falls below this range, use heart rate at 15 RPE as LTHR. If VT is higher than the range of 15 to 17, use heart rate at 17 RPE as LTHR.

Another way of estimating LTHR is from a bike time trial done either as a race or as a solo workout. This is best on a flat, out-and-back course with no stop streets and little traffic. If you do it as a

Table 3.2

VENTILATORY THRESHOLD DATA

Speed	Heart rate	RPE
15	110	8
16	118	10
17	125	12
18	135	13
19	142	14
20	147	15
21	153	17 VT
22	156	19
23	159	20

workout, mark the start-finish and turn around points, or use fixed landmarks for subsequent tests. The course length may be from 5 kilometers to 40 kilometers. The longer the course, the more accurate the results. Ride the course on a day when you are rested and there is minimal wind. Warm up well. Start your heart rate monitor as you begin the time trial, and stop it when you cross the finish line. Dividing your average heart rate for the time trial by the appropriate number in table 3.3 will estimate your LTHR.

Table 3.3

ESTIMATING LACTATE THRESHOLD HEART RATE FROM A TIME TRIAL

Distance	As race	As workout
5 km	1.10	1.04
10 km	1.07	1.02
8-10 mi	1.05	1.01
40 km	1.00	0.97

To estimate LTHR, divide average heart rate from a time trial of a distance listed here by the number in a column to the right of it, depending on whether the time trial was a race or a workout.

Training Zones

Bear in mind that the LTHR you come up with, no matter which method you use—including a lab test, is only an estimate. Retests and close monitoring of heart rate during workouts and events are necessary to more accurately estimate LTHR. With a ballpark estimate, however, you can now determine personal bike training zones. Training zones are computed by multiplying LTHR by certain percentages. By training within those boundaries, you reap specific benefits. Table 3.4 lists these percentages and the physiological gains expected from

Table 3.4

TRAINING ZONE WORKOUT TYPES AND BENEFITS

Zone	LTHR (%)	Workout type	General benefits
1	65-81	Steady ride	Rejuvenation
		Interval recoveries	Aerobic endurance
			Slow twitch muscles
2	82-88	Steady ride	Aerobic endurance
			Slow twitch muscles
3	89-93	Steady ride	Aerobic endurance
		Long intervals	Slow twitch and fast twitch type IIa muscles
4	94-99	Steady ride	Maximal aerobic endurance
		Long intervals	Anaerobic endurance
			Slow twitch and fast twitch type IIa muscles
5a	100-102	Steady ride	Maximal aerobic endurance
		Long intervals	Anaerobic endurance
			Slow twitch and fast twitch type IIa muscles
5b	103-105	Intervals	Anaerobic endurance
			Fast twitch type IIa, IIb muscles
			Aerobic capacity
5c	106+	Repetitions	Fast twitch type IIb muscles
			Anaerobic capacity
			Lactate tolerance

each zone. Note that these zones are for cycling only and not applicable to other sports. Chapters 5 and 6 provide suggested training schedules based on the periodization model and these training zones.

Measuring Progress

A heart rate monitor can help determine progress toward greater cycling fitness. It's a good idea to check progress about once a month. One way to do this is to simply repeat the lactate threshold test on a stationary bike or indoor trainer. Plot both tests on an XY graph. A shift of the posttest graphed line to the right of the pretest line indicates improving aerobic fitness. Figure 3.6 illustrates this.

Another way to check progress is to ride a standard out-and-back route, such as your LT time-trial course, at a heart rate that is 9 to 11 beats per minute less than estimated lactate threshold heart rate. This is called an aerobic time trial (ATT).

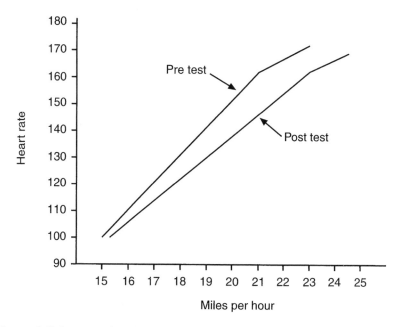

Figure 3.6 Lactate threshold heart rate tests done before and after a period of training. Fitness improvement is evident from the shift to the right of the post test.

Warm up, then ride a standard ATT course that takes 10 to 15 minutes. If your aerobic fitness is improving, the time for the ATT is faster than on a previous test. Don't expect big changes. A 2-percent shift for a fit rider is a lot. There are also many variables, such as weather, health, fatigue, mental stress, and diet that affect the results of such test, so prepare for what appears to be slipping fitness even though you can sense improvement. The human body is not a simple organism to measure.

Advanced Training

Despite alloy frame materials and fancy new components, the basic design of the bike has changed little since the 1960s. What's changed most is you. You're older and your cycling fitness may have changed in the last few years due to lots of slow, easy miles. Although this develops a great aerobic system, when it comes time for the tough stuff, such as climbing, riding into the wind, and sprinting, the legs just aren't there. So, what can you do to get them back? This chapter shows how to train for the bike fitness that you need to ride strongly, regardless of conditions. It examines your cycling-specific strengths and weaknesses, describes how to improve the weaknesses, and how to peak your fitness at the right times.

Finding Your Limits

The starting point for improving fitness is knowing what physical weaknesses are holding you back. Once you know these performance limiters, you can set your bike up in a way that produces stronger riding and decide what elements of fitness to focus training on. The following self-test will help determine what's holding your riding back and if you're ready for advanced training.

Read each statement and decide if it describes you. Circle the appropriate answer: A for agree, D for disagree. If unsure, go with your initial feeling.

Table 4.1

PERSONAL CYCLING PROFILE

A = Agree   D= Disagree

A   D   1. I'm quite lean compared with others I ride with.

A   D   2. I'm usually capable of catching other riders who are several minutes ahead.

A   D   3. I'm good at sprinting.

A   D   4. I'm capable of enduring continuous discomfort on the bike, accompanied by heavy breathing for long periods, perhaps as long as 30 to 60 minutes.

A   D   5. I'm stronger at the end of long rides than most of my training partners.

A   D   6. I can climb long hills better than most of my training partners.

A   D   7. I can spin at cadences in excess of 120 revolutions per minute without bouncing.

A   D   8. I look forward to the hills when riding.

A   D   9. I prefer long, moderate-intensity rides to short, fast ones.

A   D   10. I'm comfortable in an aerodynamic position with back flat and a low and narrow profile.

A   D   11. I have a lot of power based on my instantaneous sprint speed, vertical jump, or other indicator.

A   D   12. In relation to my riding partners, I get stronger as a ride gets longer.

A   D   13. Although I may be uncomfortable, I seldom blow up on climbs, even when the group's speed increases.

A   D   14. I can ride near my lactate threshold (heavy breathing) for long periods.

A   D   15. I comfortably use smaller gears with a higher cadence than most others I ride with.

A   D   16. In an individual time trial, with the exception of turn arounds and hills, I can stay seated the entire duration.

A   D   17. In a group sprint, I feel strong and physically capable of winning.

A   D   18. In most sports, I've been able to finish the game stronger than others.

A   D   19. When standing on a climb, I feel light and nimble on the pedals.

A   D   20. I'm confident of my endurance at the start of long rides.

Score your answers to determine your strengths and weaknesses. For each of the following sets of numbered questions, count the circled A answers and write the total in the space provided.

Totals

Endurance score—Total "agrees" for questions 5, 9, 12, 18, 20 _____

Climbing score—Total "agrees" for questions 1, 6, 8, 13, 19   _____

Sprinting score—Total "agrees" for questions 3, 7, 11, 15, 17   _____

Time-trial score—Total "agrees" for questions 2, 4, 10, 14, 16   _____

Your strengths are those with scores of 4 or 5. All the others are limiting your riding performance. The lower the score, the greater the limiter. In the rest of this chapter, when it comes to setting your bike up or deciding what to focus on in training, keep these limiters in mind.

If you don't have a strength in at least one of these cycling proficiency areas, focus on building endurance until it's a strength before training the other limiters.

BUYING THE RIGHT BIKE

If you're in the market for a new bike, getting one that fits you will make a huge difference, not only in how well you perform, but also in your comfort for those long rides. The best way to purchase a bike is to go to a reputable bike shop, one that specializes in bicycle sales and repair, and hires people who also ride. Such a shop is more likely to have bikes that fit your needs and the expertise to correctly fit you than a general sporting goods dealer or a discount store.

Buying the right bike is as much a matter of knowing yourself as it is budgeting. Although a helpful salesperson will assist with the many choices, knowing a few points in advance will make you a more informed shopper and quickly narrow the choices.

Fiftyish riders often need a bike designed with comfort upper-most in mind. We have less tolerance for jarring and the accompa-nying wear and tear on the body with tightly strung, high-perfor-mance bikes. Although steep seat-tube angles in the range of 75 to 80 degrees are often the choice of time trialists and multisport athletes, they transmit more road shock. Seat-tube angles less than 75 degrees used with a forward-angled seat post can solve this problem. Better yet, a beam bike, or frame made from titanium or carbon fiber will reduce the jarring. Mountain bikes with front-end or full suspension are also a wise choice.

Your sex has a lot to do with which bike you ultimately buy. Men have fewer problems in selecting a bike because most frames are designed to fit a man's torso-to-leg ratios. This means that when a woman finds a bike that is the right height, she is often too stretched out reaching for the handlebars. The shorter a woman is, the more critical top-tube and seat-tube lengths become. Standing less than 63 inches tall practically requires a special woman's frame or even a custom-made bike. There are some companies that make bikes designed to fit a woman's proportions. Ask your dealer for details.

Weight is an issue in picking a new bike. Weighing more than 180 pounds usually requires a heavier frame that can take the greater stresses you'll place on it. If you're a big rider, be cautious of frames weighing less than three pounds. Check the weight limit of the frame.

Remember when deciding on a new bike that getting the frame right is the most important point. You can change all other fit-related components, such as handlebar stems, crank arms, and seat posts, to improve the fit. Most dealers will happily make these changes for you, but will charge the difference for upgrades.

Dialing in Your Bike

The starting point for riding at your best under all conditions is having a bike that fits correctly. Once the bike is right, then you can develop advanced fitness more easily.

In setting up a bike to get the most from your fitness level, there are four points to consider. In order of importance, they are safety, comfort, aerodynamics, and power. The bike is fitted to your unique needs with these priorities in mind, adjusting or replacing the points where you contact it. There are small, individual fitting variances, depending on whether it's a road, mountain, or time-trial bike, and your intended use of it. The following steps will help make your bike position safe, aerodynamic, and powerful. You may need to make small adjustments for comfort.

Cleat Position

Consider your strengths and weaknesses, and how you'll use the bike. The farther forward on the shoe the cleats are, the faster you'll spin the cranks. This is beneficial for criterium racing and sprinting. Moving the cleats toward the heel of the shoe improves the application of force to the pedals and pays off when climbing hills or time trialing.

Crank Arm Length

How long is your pants inseam? If less than 31 inches, start with 170-millimeter cranks (the length is stamped on the back). If your inseam is 31 to 33 inches, your base length is 172.5-millimeter cranks. An inseam longer than 33 inches calls for a 175-millimeter crank. Modify your starting size, if needed, in the following way. If you race on the track, subtract 2.5 or 5 millimeters. Time trialists and triathletes may add 2.5 millimeters. Mountain bikers add 5 millimeters. Add no more than 2.5 millimeters at a time to avoid knee injuries. If you have nagging knee problems, try reducing the length by 2.5 millimeters. It will take your body four to six weeks to adapt to the new size. Should you change to longer cranks, be cautious with hills during this period.

Saddle Fore-Aft Position

Move the saddle forward and backward only to improve pedaling, not to change your reach to the handlebars. An incorrect reach means you need either a different-length stem (more on that later) or a different-sized bike.

To adjust the fore-aft position, sit on your bike while on an indoor trainer on a flat surface. Spin for a while to warm up and to find a comfortable position. Stop pedaling, and with the crank arms parallel to the floor, drop a plumb line from the bump just below the kneecap of your forward leg. The line should fall within a quarter of an inch forward of or behind the axle of the pedal. A line that falls forward of the axle improves spinning, and a more rearward plumb line means better climbing. Triathletes and mountain bikers typically want the saddle forward, meaning the plumb line falls slightly in front of the axle. Road racers, century, and tour riders usually prefer the saddle in the rear position with the plumb line falling directly through the axle or slightly behind.

The saddle should be parallel to the floor or tipped up slightly for most cyclists. Time trialists may want to slightly drop the nose of the saddle below parallel for comfort in the aero position.

Saddle Height

While still on the trainer with cycling shoes on, put a pedal at the 6 o'clock position, unclip that foot, and try to put your heel on the pedal without the hips rocking. The approximate neutral position is with the knee locked out straight and the heel just touching the pedal. To improve time trialing in the aerodynamic position, raise the saddle up to one-half inch higher than neutral. To improve spinning, lower the saddle until there is a slight bend in the knee. Remember that as the saddle goes up, it also moves backward, so you may need to readjust the fore-aft position. Again, be kind to your knees. As the saddle goes down, more shearing forces are placed on the underside of the kneecap. As the saddle rises, stress is placed on the back of the knee where the hamstring tendons attach.

Handlebar Height

When riding in the upright position, with a slight elbow bend, you should have a 45-degree bend at the waist, allowing you to drop your chest for a more aerodynamic position or to weight the front wheel while climbing on a mountain bike.

Stem Length

When sitting upright with a slight elbow bend, the handlebars should visually overlap the front wheel axle. If you can see the front axle beyond the handlebars, you may need a longer stem. Should the axle visually be behind the handlebars, you may need a shorter stem.

BRAIN BUCKETS

The first step in becoming a smart cyclist is realizing that riding a bike has inherent dangers associated with it. After all, on a road bike you're like a mouse in an elephant stampede. Is off-road riding better? Although there aren't any 2,000-pound behemoths on the trails frequented by mountain bikers, "end-o's"—end-over-end crashes—on rugged and fast descents can have just as devastating an effect as a collision with a car.

There are only two kinds of cyclists, regardless of whether they ride a road or mountain bike: those who have crashed and those who are going to. Is this an overly pessimistic statement about the sport? Perhaps, but according to the American Academy of Orthopaedic Surgeons there were 599,874 cycling-related accidents in 1995 that were bad enough to send someone to the emergency room of a U.S. hospital. Cycling topped the list of sport-related hospital visits. By comparison, football was down the list in fourth place with 390,180 visits—about 65 percent of cycling's toll.

Granted, there are more people on bikes than on football fields, but safety is still a major concern in cycling. Each year in the United States there are about 1,300 deaths and 140,000 others who suffer head and facial injuries while riding a bike. About half of the deaths occur in riders over the age of 14, and head injuries are the cause of death in 75 percent of these fatalities. A bike helmet can greatly reduce the chances of an accident causing a head injury or death. Unfortunately, only about 6 percent of American bicycle riders use a helmet. I urge you to always wear one when on a ride. This is not a good place to skimp on your cycling budget.

When buying a bike helmet, look for a decal on the inside indicating that it meets federal testing standards. The sticker should be from one of these organizations: the Snell Memorial Foundation, the American National Standards Institute (ANSI), or the American Society for Testing and Materials (ASTM). The Snell standards are the highest as of this writing.

Beyond the Limits

As you can see, position on the bike has a lot to do with power production and speed in turning the cranks, both concerns for past-50 cyclists. By setting your bike up considering the limiters you want to improve, for example, moving your cleats back in their slots and setting the saddle back for stronger climbing, you're well on the way to improving. The next step to improving your weaknesses is to work on them in training. Here's how to strengthen weaknesses in the areas of endurance, climbing, sprinting, and time trialing through proper workout selection. Chapters 5 and 6 will develop these advanced training components into comprehensive training programs.

Endurance for the Long Haul

The ability to keep going, even when fatigue is setting in, is critical for success in road and off-road riding. If you identified endurance as a weakness earlier in the Personal Cycling Profile, even if it wasn't your greatest weakness, your training must concentrate on improving it first and foremost. Until you have the endurance to maintain a steady pace for the whole distance, it does not matter what the other limiters are.

There are three types of endurance—cardiorespiratory, aerobic, and muscular. It is usually best if you develop them in that order, because the first, cardiorespiratory, is the most basic and the last, muscular, the most advanced. Developing endurance is much like making a three-layer cake in that each layer or type of endurance is supported by the previous one. Just as a two-layer cake isn't as deep as a three-layer, not developing all three types of endurance means shallow fitness.

Cardiorespiratory Endurance

Cardiorespiratory endurance is the type of fitness that relates to the heart (cardio) and lungs (respiratory). As you learned in chapter 1, both systems decline with disuse and, as with all other fitness parameters, decline faster if not frequently challenged. Fortunately, it's easy to challenge and improve the heart and lungs.

The heart and lungs are considered central systems. In other words, no matter what aerobic activity you do, both are stressed. The heart and lungs don't know the difference between cycling or running or swimming or any other sport that provides continuous and rhythmic movement. Cyclists typically go through a period in the late fall or early winter, following a brief time away from serious training, when they concentrate on reestablishing cardiorespiratory endurance by pursuing other sport activities. In doing this they not only rebuild the heart's ability to pump blood efficiently by increasing the size of the main chamber and maintaining the elasticity of the lungs and chest wall, but also rest from being on the bike. Such a respite helps maintain enthusiasm for riding throughout the year.

Triathletes and other riders who cross train are effectively developing their cardiorespiratory systems by participating in two or more endurance activities.

Aerobic Endurance

Once the endurance capabilities of the heart and lungs improve, the rider focuses on developing the body's ability to store and transport fuel and produce energy. This is critical to aerobic endurance and is specific to the activity, so riding a bike is necessary to fully develop it. You can't get in top aerobic shape for cycling by doing any other activity.

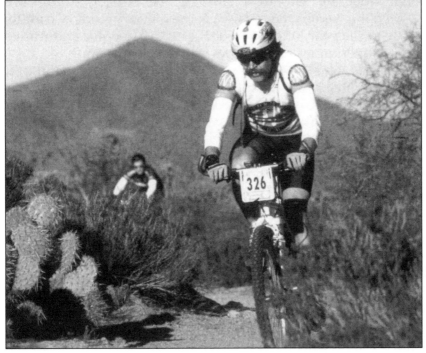

A desert race presents challenging terrain and conditions.

There are many benefits that come from aerobic endurance. All dramatically improve the ability to ride a long time. In fact, aerobic endurance is among the most trainable aspects of fitness. Some benefits that result from better aerobic fitness are the following.

- Increased capacity for storing glycogen
- Greater ability to release and transport stored body fat
- Increased capillary beds in the muscles
- Increased oxidative enzymes for burning fat
- More mitochondria—the muscles' power production centers
- Elevated aerobic capacity ($\dot{V}O_2$max)
- Preferential use of fat for fuel rather than carbohydrate

Throughout most of the training year, the cyclist should spend a great deal of time fully developing this type of endurance, for without it, nothing else is likely to improve. Developing aerobic endurance is the primary focus of training early in the year, after developing cardiovascular endurance, and is maintained throughout the riding season.

Aerobic endurance is initially improved by riding at subanaerobic heart rates. This is heart rate zones 1 to 4 as explained in chapter 3. Some coaches and athletes believe that doing even a little anaerobic training too early in the season, especially in heart rate zones 5b and 5c, is counterproductive to optimally developing aerobic fitness. Although there is no scientific evidence to support this position, it's probably best to avoid the heart rate 5 zone early in the training year when the purpose is aerobic fitness.

Long rides are the basic workout for improving aerobic endurance. By gradually increasing the duration of the longest weekly ride, your aerobic system will be stressed and forced to adapt. The physiological benefits listed previously result from gradual increases in workout time. Trying to go too far, too soon is likely to cause setbacks. The body seems incapable of absorbing great increases in duration. How much is too much? That's a difficult question to answer for all riders, but you'll certainly know when you reach it. For example, an Arizona rider recently jumped from a long ride of three hours to seven hours in a week. He was unable to ride for days after this odyssey workout, then at only a low level of intensity for several more days. The forced time off caused a loss of fitness that took a couple weeks to reacquire. Remember the rule of moderation. Keep increases small, in the range of 10 to 15 percent of your longest ride in the last six weeks.

Once you develop aerobic endurance by doing long rides, you can bring it to a peak with a few weeks of *speed-endurance intervals*. These intervals are three to six minutes with recovery periods of equal length. Include 9 to 30 minutes of these high intensity intervals within a workout. The intensity should build to the heart rate 5b zone on each. An example of a speed-endurance interval workout is four-minute intervals done five times, building to the 5b zone with 4-minute recoveries in the 1 zone. In training shorthand, this would be written as

5 × 4 minutes @ 5b (4 minutes @ 1).

Such workouts are stressful and best followed by at least 48 hours of recovery. Eight weeks of them is about all you need to build great aerobic endurance once you've achieved all that is possible with long rides. Going much beyond eight weeks increases the risk of injury, illness, overtraining, and burnout. You may not need even eight weeks to achieve a high level of fitness.

Later, this chapter explains how to peak your fitness several times within a year. It may be necessary to rebuild aerobic endurance to high levels with intervals for each peak.

Muscular Endurance

As with aerobic endurance, muscular endurance is specific to cycling; it's not fully developed by any other activity. This is a high level of endurance that relates to the muscles' ability to cope with the fatigue associated with the buildup of lactate and the depletion of glycogen. The purpose of delaying the onset of this type of fatigue is to allow the cyclist to ride farther and faster before the muscles begin to scream for relief.

Although muscular endurance is improved simply from riding a lot of miles at a moderate intensity, it is optimally developed with three types of workouts—tempo rides, cruise intervals, and threshold rides. These workouts moderately stress the body's ability to remove lactate from the blood and to buffer its fatiguing effects, while teaching the muscles to rely more heavily on fat for fuel as they spare glycogen. Good muscular endurance means being able to maintain a high speed for a long time. This type of fitness grows from work near the lactate threshold and is incorporated throughout most of the year. It is an important factor in outstanding performance. If you want to be a strong rider, muscular endurance is what you need.

Tempo rides are the first step in boosting muscular endurance. Extended efforts of 20 minutes or more with heart rate in the 3 zone are an effective way to start the long buildup to greater muscular endurance. Four to eight weeks of tempo training is all you need before progressing to the next level of development. Once past this initial stage of improving muscular endurance, avoid the 3 zone. An example of a tempo workout is

20 minutes @ 3.

Cruise intervals are the next step in muscular endurance boosting. Following a thorough warm-up, complete three to five work intervals of 6- to 12-minutes duration each. Heart rate should rise into the 4 and 5a zones during each of these. The cruise interval starts as soon as you begin riding fast, *not* when you achieve the 4 zone. The reason for this is that the muscles are receiving adequate stress to cause a training effect, even though the heart has not caught up with the demands of the first few minutes. It may take a couple minutes to reach the 4 zone on the first interval. On subsequent efforts, heart rate will respond more quickly. Keep recovery intervals short, two or three minutes, with heart rates dropping into the 1 zone, to keep a little lactate in the blood and continued demand on the aerobic system. Most riders do cruise intervals once or twice a week early in the year, followed by 36 to 48 hours of recovery. An example of a cruise interval workout is

4 × 8 minutes @ 4 to 5a (2 minutes @ 1).

The combined work interval time in a single workout is usually 18 to 60 minutes, but sometimes, as in recovery weeks, as little as 9 to 15 minutes of cruise intervals is effective for maintaining this kind of fitness. Although riders usually do cruise intervals on a flat course, a common variation is to do them on a long, slight uphill grade (2 to 4 percent) to simultaneously develop climbing strength.

Do *threshold rides* after you have developed a substantial level of fitness with cruise intervals. When you can comfortably complete 30 to 40 minutes or more of cruise intervals, it's time to start threshold rides by riding continuously for 20 minutes or more in the heart rate 4 and 5a zones. Every couple weeks add another five minutes until you reach about 40 minutes. Do these on a flat or gently rolling course. Ride in an aerodynamic position and pay close attention to your breathing. You should stay right on the edge of labored breathing. By the way, if labored breathing is what you experience when you are in the upper 4 or 5a heart rate zones, then your lactate threshold heart rate determined earlier is probably correct. An example of a threshold ride is

30 minutes @ 4 or 5a.

A variation for the highly fit cyclist is to include two or three of these 20-minute threshold efforts within a single workout, with 5 to 10 minutes of recovery between them. An example of such a ride is

2 × 20 minutes @ 4-5a (10 minutes @ 1).

The threshold ride is a little more stressful than cruise intervals due to its length, and you should limit them to once a week. You will probably need at least 48 hours to recover.

Climbing With the Mountain Goats

Cyclists are more concerned with climbing than any other aspect of fitness, and for good reason, as hills are the greatest challenge in riding a bike. An adage among bike racers is, "If you can't climb, you can't race." Even if you live in the flat regions of the United States, such as coastal Florida or Kansas, training for better climbing will make you a stronger rider on the flats.

It's difficult to separate all the physiological components of climbing. Certainly cardiorespiratory, aerobic, and muscular endurance all play an important role in conquering hills. If one

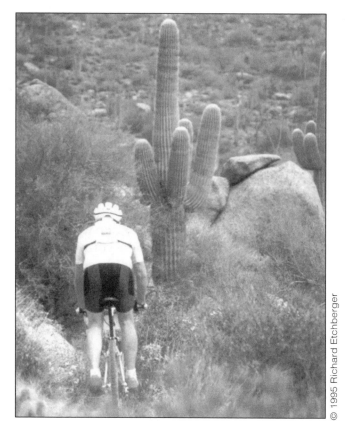

© 1995 Richard Etchberger

Oracle Ridge, Tucson, Arizona

of these is weak, you climb poorly. Assuming all types of endurance are well developed, however, how can you best train to improve weak climbing?

Climbing and Body Weight

Getting over long and steep hills is largely a function of your strength-to-body weight ratio. As strength goes up and excess body weight goes down, climbing improves. Let's look at weight first. The best climbers in the professional peloton typically weigh less than two pounds per inch of height. Most of the nonclimbers in the pro field are 2.2 to 2.3 pounds per inch. There are no active pros at 2.5 pounds per inch or greater. Climbing favors those who are lean. It's been estimated that every extra kilogram of fat (2.2 pounds) adds three seconds in a one-kilometer climb (.62 miles) on a moderate grade of about 5 percent.

We've all known big riders who could climb, however. How do they manage to stay up front on hills, even though they don't fit the climbers' body mold? The Spanish pro and five-time winner of the Tour de France, Miguel Indurain, is a good example of this. At the peak of his career he could stay with the small, lightweight climbers when he needed to, even though he was six-foot, two-inches tall and weighed 172 pounds. That's more than 2.3 pounds per inch, big by world-class cycling standards. Indurain and other big riders who can climb must have something else going for them—great leg-extension strength.

Leg-extension strength is the ability to straighten the hip, knee, and ankle against a heavy load. Strength increases in this critical cycling movement can overcome a large body weight. The best way to develop this strength is to ride in the hills a lot, but that may also be hard on knees that aren't prepared for such training. An alternative, which is quite effective, is weightlifting, especially doing such exercises as the half squat, step-up, and leg press.

New riders who need to improve their climbing typically attack the problem on two fronts by losing excess body weight and increasing leg-extension strength. Set reasonable goals for both at the start of the training season, and monitor them regularly throughout the early weeks of annual training. Chapter 8 will help you develop an effective strength program. Weight loss is best done slowly—a process in which you shed one or two pounds of fat weekly for a month or so, followed by a month of maintenance before attempting to lose more fat. Small decreases in daily food intake of 200 to 300 calories while maintaining aerobic and strength training are often all you need. This is the number of calories in one small piece of pie or cake or 15 french fries.

Climbing Skills

Climbing is also a matter of skill. As you approach a long or steep hill, keep the speed high without shifting. Allow momentum to carry you up the first few yards, then shift to an easier gear just before the free ride ends. It's probably best that the gear combination you select to climb in keeps your cadence fairly low, perhaps in the range of 60 to 70 revolutions per minute. This better sustains power while maintaining low blood lactate levels than a gear that requires a high cadence. Such a low cadence while climbing demands a great deal of leg-extension strength and healthy knees. If this puts excessive stress on the knees, or you feel like you're bogging down, use an easier gear that permits more spinning.

Should you stand or stay seated on long hills? On the road, big riders (2.2 pounds per inch or more) are usually better off staying on the saddle, but small riders are often better standing. Women are generally advised to stand while climbing, as they have a greater proportion of their body weight below the waist, hence less dead upper body weight to support than men. Alternating standing and sitting will shift the strain on certain muscle groups to others, allowing a momentary rest before resuming the preferred position. Mountain bikers are usually better off staying seated, adding weight to the front wheel to keep it from coming off the ground. If seated climbing bothers your knees, predominantly stand on the hills regardless of the optimal style for your size and event.

When standing on a road bike, grasp the brake hoods and straighten your back while getting out of the saddle on a downstroke. Don't lean on the handlebars, but rather put your weight over the pedals as you pull against the brake on the same side as the descending foot. The side-to-side rocking of the bike is a subtle movement, not exaggerated. Get the feeling that you're running on the pedals.

When climbing in the saddle on the road, sit back, straighten your back, and hold the handlebars near the stem. This allows the full use of the back and butt muscles in pushing through the top of the stroke. Dropping the heel at the top of the stroke adds more power. Relax the upper body, especially the hands, as much as possible so you don't waste energy.

Seated climbing on a mountain bike is different. On steep climbs, which are common on trails, sit forward on the saddle and lean on the handlebars by bending the elbows. This keeps the front wheel from coming up. Emphasize the downstroke all the way through the 6 o'clock position while pulling up on the recovery pedal. Try to maintain even tension on the chain throughout 360 degrees of the pedal stroke.

Climbing Workouts

There are lots of possibilities for workouts that involve hills. Here are three that will improve your climbing.

Moderate hills. Ride a course with several climbs of up to a 6-percent grade. This is about the same grade as an interstate overpass that takes two or three minutes to climb. Stay seated when climbing these hills, focusing on a smooth and even pedal stroke and little body movement. Keep your cadence at 50 revolutions per minute or more. Go no higher than the heart rate 5a zone.

Long hills. Find a long hill with a 4- to 6-percent grade that takes four to eight minutes to climb. Repeat this hill several times until you've accumulated 20 to 30 minutes of climbing with coast-down recoveries after each. Ride with cadence at 50 to 70 revolutions per minute. Raise heart rate into the 5a zone on each climb.

Steep hills. Do repeats on a short, steep hill of 8-percent grade or more that takes 90 seconds to 2 minutes to climb. For century riders, road racers, and triathletes, 8 percent is the highest grade you need, as these are usually the steepest hills on state and federal highways. Mountain bikers should find a steeper grade off road. Climb in and out of the saddle, alternating positions and experimenting with technique.

Powerful Sprinting

There's no greater thrill in cycling than winning a sprint, whether it's going for the finish line with another racer or sprinting for the city limits sign with friends. A weakness in this category means you're spit out the back when the group winds up for the big finish. It also makes you easy pickings for that dog on your favorite route. Sprinting can also make a difference when a driver overestimates the yellow light at an intersection just as you're starting through.

Physics of Sprinting

Power is the obvious talent of good sprinters. Although we often talk about power in cycling, few really know what it means. In physics, power is the rate at which work is done. To put it another way, power is force divided by time. In language that cyclists use, power is the ability to quickly turn the pedals while in a high gear.

What this means is that there are two qualities necessary for good sprinting—strength and leg speed. Having one without the other is useless for a sprint. Cycling strength, as discussed in the earlier section on climbing, is the ability to extend the hip, knee, and ankle. Building strength for sprinting is just like building strength for climbing, at least when it comes to weight training (more on weight training in chapter 8). The difference is in leg speed.

The best sprinters have the ability to quickly turn the cranks. In low gears, such as 39 by 19, they may be able to spin up to 140 revolutions per minute or more. When most of us try that, we begin to bounce on the saddle at much lower cadences. There are two possible causes for this bouncing. The first has to do with genetics. The best sprinters typically have

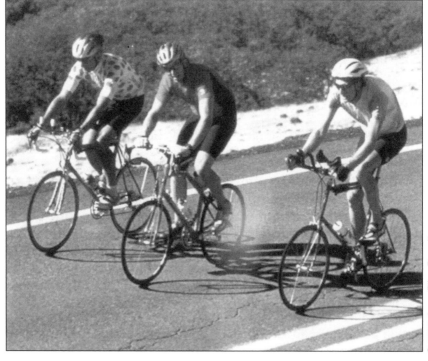

© 1997 Anne Flinn Powell

Training partners help you push your limits.

lots of fast twitch muscle, which contracts quickly but fatigues fast. Those with great endurance, but lacking sprinting ability, may be blessed with an abundance of slow twitch muscle, which contracts slowly but is resistant to fatigue, and little of the fast twitch type. In other words, great sprinters are born to sprint. However, don't lose hope; there is another way to improve leg speed.

The second cause of weak spinning ability has to do with economy. Economy is the ability to recruit and relax muscles at the right times and is highly trainable. For example, consider only the actions of the quadriceps muscle on the front of the thigh and the hamstring muscle on the back of the thigh during a sprint. To push the pedal down, your central nervous system activates, or recruits, the quadriceps. When this muscle contracts, the knee straightens out. At the bottom of the pedal stroke, you must allow the quadriceps to relax at the precise time the hamstring is pulling the pedal back and up. If the nervous system tells the quadriceps to relax milliseconds too late, the result you experience is bouncing on the saddle. In other words, at the bottom of the stroke, the quadriceps is still trying to extend the knee, even though the pedal can't go any lower. Because the pedal can't move farther down—the crank arm can't be stretched—your body moves up. You come off the saddle.

You can change this by teaching the nervous system to use the muscles in precise harmony. Even if your parents gave you all the genes necessary to be a sprinter, this is still something you must continually work on. Here are workouts to improve your leg speed and economy. Heart rate has no significance for any of them, so a heart rate monitor is unnecessary. They are listed in a progressive order, with the most basic ones first, laying the groundwork for the advanced skills.

Sprint Workouts

Spin-ups. After warming up, start in a low gear, such as 39 by 16; spin at a faster-than-normal cadence for 10 seconds. Then shift to a lower gear, such as 39 by 17, and spin at a still higher cadence for 10 seconds. Finally, shift lower one more time, and spin at the highest cadence you can hold for 10 seconds. If you bounce in the last 10 seconds, slow leg speed slightly until the bouncing stops. Recover for 60 to 90 seconds, and repeat up to eight times or until leg speed noticeably drops off. On the road, do these on a slight downhill or with a tailwind. In the winter, this is a perfect indoor workout for a trainer or rollers. You can do spin-ups several times a week.

Isolated leg. On a slight downhill or with a tailwind, do 90 percent of the work with one leg as the other goes along for the ride. Spin in an easy gear while attempting to smooth out the dead spots at the top and bottom of the stroke. Change legs when fatigue sets in. Indoors, you can do these on a trainer by taking one foot out of the pedals and placing it on a chair or stool while the other does all the work.

Fixed gear. Riding a bike with a single gear combination and no freewheel has gone out of style in the last 10 years. That's too bad, because using such a bike, especially in the early stages of the annual training cycle, is an excellent way to develop smoother pedaling at high cadence. The fixed gear will also improve climbing strength and cornering skills. If you were a serious cyclist in the 1960s or 1970s, you've probably used a fixed-gear bike and may still own one. If not, have a local bike shop set up an old bike for you as a fixed gear; then ride it once or twice a week early in the training season on a flat course. Stay away from big hills. The gear combination you select for this bike should allow you to maintain a cadence slightly higher than normal when riding comfortably on a flat road. This is generally in the range of 39 to 42 by 15 to 19. Use caution when first starting to use a fixed-gear bike, as you'll have to change old habits, such as standing on the pedals to stretch and cornering with an extreme lean.

Form sprints. On the road, with a slight tailwind or downhill, complete several 8- to 15-second sprints with the focus on form, rather than power. Stand the first few seconds as you build speed. During this jump, hold the handlebars deep in the drops and pull on the same side as the pedal you're driving down. Initially, your weight should stay back over the rear wheel to keep it down. As speed increases, move the hips forward with the elbows bent to maintain an aerodynamic position. At the bottom of the stroke have a slight bend in the knees to maintain constant torque on the chain. Always keep your head up so you can see where you're going. Once speed is at the top end, practice sitting and standing on alternate sprints. Experiment with positions. Try different gearing combinations. Practice shifting on the fly. Which is your greatest form weakness? Focus on that. Recover for five minutes after each form sprint, and complete 6 to 10 of them. If form becomes sloppy, stop the workout. Remember, the emphasis of this workout is on form and finesse, not fitness. These are best done alone.

Match sprints. With a training partner or group, do several competition sprints for designated landmarks. Include both short, 10-second, and long, 30-second, efforts. Although these are maximum effort sprints, don't get sloppy. Continue using the same technique refined with the form sprints. Recover for three to five minutes after each sprint.

Unlimited Time Trialing

In road racing, the time trial is called the race of truth because there's no team to hide behind, no pack on which to draft, and no support. You're out there alone, finding out who you *really* are as a rider. The same goes for mountain bike racing; it's sometimes called a "time trial on trails." Of course, for amateur triathletes and duathletes, time trialing is what racing is all about. For the recreational cyclist, good time-trial ability means stronger cycling and riding at the front of the group instead of off the back and trying to catch up. The time trial is the ultimate test of the cyclist.

Time trialing is 80-percent body, 10-percent brain, and 10-percent bike. Let me explain those in reverse order.

There's little doubt that having the right bike makes for faster time trials. How much faster depends on how much you are willing to spend to buy time. For example, it's been estimated that while riding at 25 miles per hour on a 40-kilometer course, aero bars costing about $65 will save 3 minutes, 21 seconds. That's 32 cents per second. Pretty cheap, especially considering that a disc wheel at about $580 will cut another 58 seconds from your time. That's more like $10 a second. This is just scratching the surface. You could purchase aero-bar-end shifters, an aero-drinking system, aero helmet, 18-millimeter tires, and a deep-rim front wheel at a combined cost of $570 and further reduce 40-kilometer time by 4 minutes, 21 seconds: another $2.18 per second.

So, a fast bike obviously is one way to be good at time trialing. The second way is to train your brain. We require patience, something we older riders are usually good at, to time trial well. Learning to hold back at the start and pace yourself is paramount. If you pace the race correctly, you cross the finish line just as you run out of gas. Pacing skill comes from lots of practice at reading your body and knowing how to use a heart rate monitor.

The most important part of the time-trial puzzle is the body. The best bike in the world and the patience of Job won't make you a good time trialist if fitness is lacking. Time-trial fitness requires two components—endurance and strength. If this sounds familiar, that's because we covered it earlier under muscular endurance. Remember that there are three key workouts for muscular endurance, and they also apply to time-trial training. The workouts are tempo rides, cruise intervals, and threshold rides. In review, here are examples of those workouts.

- Tempo ride 20 minutes @ 3
- Cruise intervals 4 × 8 minutes @ 4-5a (2 minutes @ 1)
- Threshold ride 30 minutes @ 4-5a

These workouts have a moderate to moderately high stress level associated with them, depending on the duration of the fast-riding part of the workout, so they are possible to do frequently throughout the year. Cruise intervals, in fact, are the only type of interval workout that you may do year-round. What most of us have called intervals over the years, the gut-wrenching, go-hard-till-you-drop efforts, are best done infrequently, if at all.

Peaking When It Counts

Once you have attained a high level of fitness by improving your weakness, whether it's endurance, climbing, sprinting, or time trialing, what must you do to maintain it? If peaking for an important race or other event such as a century or tour, how can you rest without losing fitness?

You can find the answers to these questions in a study

conducted a few years ago at the University of Illinois in Chicago by Dr. Robert C. Hickson. In the first 10 weeks of his 25-week study, the subjects completed weekly sessions of running or riding stationary bikes with workouts similar to the muscular-endurance workouts described previously. On one day they trained for 40 minutes, including a threshold ride, and the next day each completed cruise intervals of six 5-minute efforts with 2-minute recoveries. Heart rates were about 90 percent of maximum in each case, or about at lactate threshold, which you'll recall is effective for improving fitness. These workouts alternated for six days followed by a day off— 10 tough weeks, needless to say.

After this initial 10-week period in which the subjects' fitness rose significantly, they were divided into three sub-groups for the next 15 weeks. One group reduced *frequency* (how often they worked out) by a third, another cut back on workout *time* by a third, and the last decreased *intensity* by a third. With each group, the other two components of training remained constant. Figure 4.1 is adapted from this study and shows what happened to aerobic capacity ($\dot{V}O_2$max) when the subjects were tested at 5-week intervals during the following 15-week period.

It's evident that when you reduce the frequency or time of riding once you have attained a high level of fitness, there is no

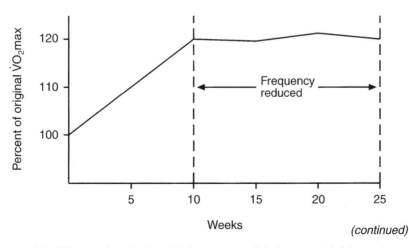

a

(continued)

Figure 4.1 Effects of reducing (a) frequency, (b) time, and (c) intensity on aerobic capacity following a 10-week training period

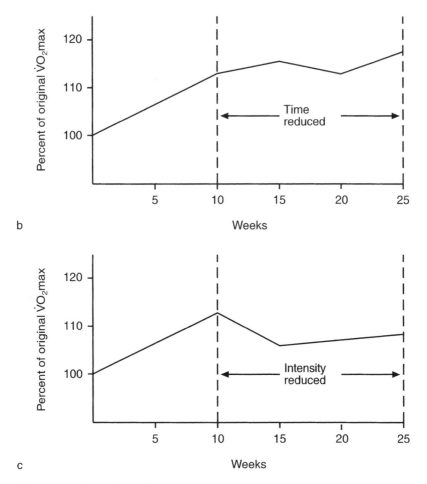

b

c

Figure 4.1 *(continued)*

From Hickson, R.C., et al. 1985. Reduced training intensities and loss of aerobic power, endurance, and cardiac growth. *Journal of Applied Physiology* 58: 497. Reprinted by permission.

appreciable change in fitness as measured by aerobic capacity. In fact, the study suggests that fitness may even improve from decreasing frequency and time. When intensity decreases, however, there is a significant drop in fitness as determined by aerobic capacity.

What this means for you is that when it's time to reach a physiological peak for an important event, you can best maintain fitness while resting by cutting back on the frequency and time of workouts and keeping the intensity high. The next two chapters suggest training schedules for different types of events that employ this principle.

5

Testing Your Limits

At first, it is the distance. How many miles can you ride in a few hours or a few days? Later, it is the speed. How fast can you ride a formerly intimidating distance? The typical events in which we choose to test ourselves are 100-mile century rides, multiday tours, and across-the-country rides. They are appealing because they challenge us mentally and physically to become more than we are now. In some deep, dark corner of our minds is that nagging thought that if we can only accomplish that distance or that speed, we'll be real cyclists. Even though we know that's silly, the self-challenging thoughts persist. You *must* go for it.

The common denominator for all these challenges is endurance. You must be able to go the distance before thinking about going fast. The previous chapter told you about the three types of endurance—cardiorespiratory, aerobic, and muscular. You need all these in vast quantities to tackle any long-duration event. The first two types are easy to develop, the third, muscular endurance, is tougher to achieve, but definitely necessary.

After endurance, the second most important fitness need is strength to get you over the hills, assuming there will be some on the route. Of course, there are a few totally flat challenges, such as the Hancock Horizontal Hundred, a century ride near Findlay, Ohio. For these, strength isn't as much of an issue.

Just get your endurance up. Most, however, have a least a few hills to challenge more than your endurance, like the Bicycle Ride Across Georgia (BRAG). Then there are the rides for which strength is every bit as important as endurance, like Ride the Rockies in Colorado, which includes six days of mountain passes with peaks higher than 10,000 feet elevation.

This chapter will teach you how to prepare for such challenges and offer guidelines for building endurance and strength before peaking at the right time. Successfully finishing one of these tests of your limits requires more than physical fitness. You also need a plan for pacing, nutrition, clothing, and equipment. A misshift in any of these vital areas could mean the end of your venture. All are addressed here.

Century Challenge

A 100-mile ride is a rite of passage in the cycling world. Most cyclists don't consider themselves complete riders until they've done a century. Once they've gone the distance, thoughts nearly always turn to doing one faster the next time. Breaking five hours, requiring a 20-mile per hour average, is a common goal for experienced century riders. Either of these, completing a first century or a doing personal best time for the distance, is a big challenge and should not be taken lightly.

Goal—Go the Distance

Preparing to finish your first century means increasing the length of your longest ride every few weeks. The long ride is far more important than the weekly volume or total time on the bike. Putting in lots of miles every week will do little more than make you tired when it's time for the all-important long ride.

If you do it correctly, the weekly long ride not only will increase all three types of endurance, but also will serve as a dress rehearsal for the century for which you're training. The idea is to make it as close as you can to the expected conditions. Start by selecting a course for these rides that is similar to the century. The entry form will often describe the hills or provide a course profile. If it will be a ride on rolling terrain, select such a course for your longest weekly ride. If it's table-top flat, train on a flat route.

Next, find a training partner preparing for the same goal, or better yet, a group of training partners. Because you'll be doing the century with other riders, you want to experience the same thing in training. Practice drafting and working in a pace line, just as you'll do in the century.

Planning to Finish

For most people, Saturday is often the best day for a long training ride, because if there's bad weather that day or a scheduling conflict comes up, you can move the ride back a day to Sunday. If you schedule it for Sunday and something gets in the way, you may not be able to get it in at all.

Your training goal in preparing for a first century is to ride four to four-and-a-half hours two weeks before the big day. Starting from your longest ride of the last two weeks, add 30 minutes each week until you achieve this time. Don't, however, take a straight-line approach to the goal time. That's likely to get you overtrained and burned out. You'll also get there too quickly, which means you won't fully develop your endurance. Table 5.1 offers a suggested schedule that ratchets the time of

Table 5.1

WEEKLY PROGRESSION OF LONG RIDES IN PREPARING FOR A CENTURY

Period 1		Period 2		Period 3	
Week 25	1:00	Week 21	1:30	Week 17	2:00
Week 24	1:30	Week 20	2:00	Week 16	2:30
Week 23	2:00	Week 19	2:30	Week 15	3:00
Week 22	1:00	Week 18	1:15	Week 14	1:30
Period 4		**Period 5**		**Period 6**	
Week 13	2:30	Week 9	3:00	Week 5	3:30
Week 12	3:00	Week 8	3:30	Week 4	4:00
Week 11	3:30	Week 7	4:00	Week 3	4:30
Week 10	1:45	Week 6	2:00	Week 2	2:15

*All times in hours:minutes.

the long ride up over several weeks. Although this ratcheting takes time, it will build a solid endurance base and plenty of long-distance riding experience.

To find the right period for you to start, look for your longest ride of the last two weeks in the second week of the six periods listed on table 5.1. The first week of that period is the one with which you should begin. For example, if your longest ride of the last two weeks is two hours, you would start training in period 2 because week 20 is a two-hour ride.

Using a calendar, count backward the number of weeks indicated as your starting week from the date of the century. In the example, you would start training 21 weeks before the century. This will allow one week at the end to taper and fully rest (more on that later).

Do the weekly long ride mostly in the heart rate 2 and 3 zones. Try to avoid the 5 zone, even on hills, because that would result in accumulating lactate throughout the ride and in premature fatigue. Gear selection is critical. If the course is hilly, you want to have a third, and smaller, chain ring installed. Although this is sometimes called a granny gear for obvious reasons, don't be put off by the cute name. Almost everyone in the century will have one on their bike too.

Weekly Workouts

The long ride is not enough training to get you ready for the century. As you learned in chapter 3, there is a minimum number of weekly workouts necessary to improve fitness. To complete a century, it's best to ride four or five times a week with two days off, sandwiching the long ride to make sure you're rested before and recovered after. The other rides should include one for aerobic maintenance with heart rates in the 2 and 3 zones, one hilly ride in all zones to build strength, and the remaining workouts as recovery rides in the 1 zone. Table 5.2 provides a suggested weekly training routine.

Goal—Go the Distance Faster

Having broken through the psychological barrier by completing a century, you're probably eager to know how quickly you can cover 100 miles the next time. Assuming you did your previous century just to finish and rode well within your limits,

Table 5.2

WEEKLY TRAINING ROUTINES TO COMPLETE A CENTURY RIDE

Buildup weeks

Monday	60- to 90-min maintenance ride in 2 and 3 zones on a rolling course, staying in saddle on hills
Tuesday	45- to 60-min recovery ride in 1 zone on a flat course, keeping cadence comfortably high, or day off if tired or unmotivated to ride
Wednesday	60 to 90 min on a hilly course in all zones
Thursday	45- to 60-min recovery ride in 1 zone on a flat course, keeping cadence comfortably high
Friday	Day off
Saturday	Long ride in 2 and 3 zones. Dress rehearsal for century
Sunday	Day off

Recovery weeks

Monday	45- to 60-min maintenance ride in 2 and 3 zones on a rolling course, staying in saddle on hills
Tuesday	Day off
Wednesday	45 to 60 min on a hilly course in all zones
Thursday	30- to 45-min recovery ride in 1 zone on a flat course, keeping cadence comfortably high, or day off if tired or unmotivated to ride
Friday	Day off
Saturday	Long ride in 2 and 3 zones. Dress rehearsal for century
Sunday	Day off

Week of century ride

Monday	30- to 45-min recovery ride in 1 zone on a flat course, keeping cadence comfortably high
Tuesday	Day off
Wednesday	30 to 45 min on a hilly course in all zones
Thursday	Day off
Friday	30- to 45-min recovery ride in 1 zone on a flat course, keeping cadence comfortably high
Saturday	Day off
Sunday	Century ride

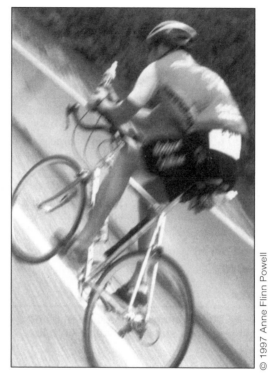

© 1997 Anne Flinn Powell

Include hill training to build strength for a time-trial effort.

it's reasonable to expect a 5- to 15-percent improvement in time on the next one.

To go faster, you need greater muscular endurance. The cruise intervals workout described in chapter 4 is perfect for developing this type of fitness. In doing this workout, you repeat long intervals with short recoveries between them. An example of a cruise interval workout for the century is four rides of six minutes with two-minute recoveries. On each interval the heart rate rises into the 4 and 5a zones. The interval starts as soon as you begin high-effort pedaling, *not* when you achieve the 4 zone. Table 5.3 lays out a suggested progression for cruise intervals. Notice that you do some on a moderate hill to create greater leg strength. Rest after each interval, in this case, by coasting down the hill while keeping your legs turning to aid recovery. If there are no hills where you

Table 5.3

WEEKLY PROGRESSION OF CRUISE INTER- VALS IN PREPARING FOR A CENTURY

Period 1

Week 13	4 × 6:00 (2:00 RI), flat
Week 12	3 × 6:00 (3:00 RI), hill
Week 11	5 × 6:00 (2:00 RI), flat
Week 10	3 × 6:00 (3:00 RI), flat

Period 2

Week 9	5 × 8:00 (3:00 RI), flat
Week 8	4 × 6:00 (3:00 RI), hill
Week 7	5 × 10:00 (3:00 RI), flat
Week 6	3 × 6:00 (3:00 RI), flat

Period 3

Week 5	4 × 6:00 (3:00 RI), hill
Week 4	5 × 12:00 (3:00 RI), flat
Week 3	5 × 6:00 (3:00 RI), hill
Week 2	3 × 6:00 (3:00 RI), flat

*All times in minutes; RI = recovery interval; "hill" means do the workout on a slight grade of about 4%.

live, do cruise intervals into a head wind on the days that hills are suggested.

The reason for doing cruise intervals is to increase the speed at which you can ride when near your lactate threshold. As lactate threshold (LT) speed increases, the speeds at all efforts slightly higher and lower also increase. Because you complete a fast century mostly in the heart rate 3 zone, 10 beats per minute or so below LT, you're able to ride faster as a result.

The other important piece in training for a fast century is pacing practice, or tempo training. At the start of a century, it's easy to go too fast thinking you have plenty of energy only to crash and burn a few hours later. Discovering the proper speed and becoming used to it will help prevent this. You do tempo work on the long rides suggested in table 5.1. Do the tempo ride exactly as you'll do the century, alone or in a pace line with other riders. Make these dress rehearsals in every possible way, including the clothing you wear, and the nutritional products and equipment you use. We highly recommend Aero bars for a fast century attempt.

During these workouts observe both heart rate and speed. Ride at goal speed using your heart rate as a governor. When riding in a pace line and pulling, as your heart rises into the high 4 zone, pull out and let the next rider take over. Avoid going into the 5 zone. If riding alone, attempt to stay in the 3 zone throughout the workout. If you're unable to stay below these heart rate limits, you must slow the speed, regardless of your goal. As muscular endurance improves from the cruise intervals, speed in the 3 and 4 zones will also improve.

Planning to Go Fast

Planning for a fast century is a little more complex than planning to finish one, as there's more to accomplish and the risk of overtraining rises considerably from the higher intensities of training. Start planning by counting 9 to 13 weeks backward from the week of the century, which is called week 1. Thirteen weeks is optimal for most, but if your muscular endurance is already high, nine weeks will do. More than 13 weeks of this intense training is likely to cause burnout.

By the time you start this final 9- to 13-week buildup to a fast century, your long ride should already be at least three hours. Table 5.1 takes you through the progression of long rides, which you now ride as goal-paced tempo workouts. Blend them in weekly with the cruise interval training of table 5.3. Do the long tempo rides on a course similar to that of the goal century.

Weekly Workouts

In addition to the cruise intervals and long tempo rides, it's a good idea to include hill training to build the necessary strength for a time-trial effort and for the hills you will encounter. Even if the course is flat, doing hill or head wind training will make you a stronger rider and better able to attain the goal time you've set. Table 5.4 offers a suggested routine for training in the buildup and recovery weeks and the week of the century.

Table 5.4

Buildup weeks

Monday	60- to 90-min maintenance ride in 2 and 3 zones on a rolling course, staying in saddle on hills
Tuesday	60- to 90-min cruise interval workout
Wednesday	45- to 60-min recovery ride in 1 zone on a flat course, keeping cadence comfortably high
Thursday	60 to 90 min on a hilly course in all zones
Friday	45- to 60-min recovery ride in 1 zone on a flat course, keeping cadence comfortably high
Saturday	Tempo ride in 2 to 4 zones if riding with a group, 3 zone if alone. Dress rehearsal for century
Sunday	Day off

Recovery weeks

Monday	45- to 60-min maintenance ride in 2 and 3 zones on a rolling course, staying in saddle on hills
Tuesday	60-min cruise interval workout
Wednesday	Day off
Thursday	45- to 60-min maintenance ride in 2 and 3 zones on a rolling course, staying in saddle on hills
Friday	Day off
Saturday	Long ride in 2 and 3 zones only
Sunday	Day off

Week of century ride

Monday	45- to 60-min maintenance ride in 2 and 3 zones on a rolling course, staying in saddle on hills
Tuesday	60-min cruise interval workout
Wednesday	Day off
Thursday	45-min maintenance ride in 2 and 3 zones on a rolling course, staying in saddle on hills
Friday	Day off
Saturday	30-min ride in 1 zone on a flat course, keeping cadence comfortably high
Sunday	Century ride

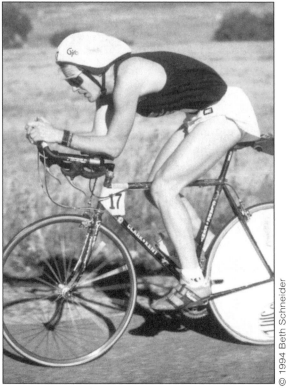

Triathlete on a Clark/Kent bike at the 1994 Coors Light Biathlon.

It's important that you closely observe the recovery weeks when training for a personal best century time. Because it's possible that recovery every fourth week is not frequent enough, you may need to follow the training pattern in table 5.5, with recovery weeks occurring every third week. You'll know whether you need a change to three-week periods if by the third week of a four-week period you feel exceptionally tired and find it difficult to complete the suggested training in tables 5.1 and 5.3.

100-Mile Tips

In preparing for a century, either a first or a fast, there are scores of details, many of which mean the difference between success and failure. Here are a few of the most important tips to help you achieve your goal.

Table 5.5

WEEKLY PROGRESSION OF CRUISE INTERVALS AND TEMPO RIDES IN PREPARING FOR A FAST CENTURY

Period 1

Week 13	4 × 6 min (2 min RI), flat
	2:30 tempo ride
Week 12	5 × 6 min (3 min RI), hill
	3:00 tempo ride
Week 11	3 × 6 min (3 min RI), flat
	1:30 tempo ride

Period 2

Week 10	5 × 8 min (3 min RI), flat
	3:00 tempo ride
Week 9	4 × 6 min (3 min RI), hill
	3:30 tempo ride
Week 8	3 × 6 min (3 min RI), flat
	1:45 tempo ride

Period 3

Week 7	5 × 10 min (3 min RI), flat
	3:30 tempo ride
Week 6	4 × 6 min (3 min RI), hill
	4:00 tempo ride
Week 5	3 × 6 min (3 min RI), flat
	2:00 tempo ride

Period 4

Week 4	5 × 12 min (3 min RI), flat
	4:00 tempo ride
Week 3	5 × 6 min (3 min RI), hill
	4:30 tempo ride
Week 2	3 × 6 min (3 min RI), flat
	2:15 tempo ride

*Based on recovery every third week.
**All times in hours:minutes; RI = recovery interval; "hill" means do the workout on a slight grade of about 4%.

The day before the century is a last chance to get everything ready. Check your bike to make sure everything is tight, properly adjusted, and ready. Just as important as the bike is your body. Drink fluids, especially water, frequently. If you've done it right, the day before will include trips to the bathroom every couple hours, and you'll be up once or twice during the night for the same reason. Also on the day before, slightly reduce the fat and protein and eat more carbohydrates, especially from nutrient-dense sources such as fruits and vegetables. Don't eat more than you normally would. Before going to bed, lay out all the clothes you'll wear and items to carry the next day. Fill bottles and put them in the refrigerator or pack them in ice if staying in a hotel.

On the morning of the century get up at least two hours before the start and have a breakfast of about 400 calories, mostly carbohydrate. This is critical, and you should practice it regularly before long rides to find out what works best. In a recent century, a first-time rider passed out 80 miles into the event and later wondered why. Although he was hydrating and eating adequately during the ride, he didn't fill his energy stores before starting, choosing to ride on an empty stomach instead. The crash resulted in an unfulfilled dream and a broken wrist.

How much is 400 calories? Here's a rough idea. A large banana or apple is about 100 calories. A serving of toast with a tablespoon of jam is about 100 calories. One ounce of cereal with skim milk provides another 100 calories. A cup of orange juice adds 100 calories. Chapter 9 offers more detailed advice on diet.

As a mental approach to the century, think of it as four 25-mile rides. Many riders find breaking it up this way into manageable blocks makes it easier to handle. Ride just as you did on the long rides. Change hand positions frequently and stretch regularly while still on the bike.

Fueling on the bike is the single most important success factor other than training. Use a sports drink every 15 minutes so you finish a 16-ounce bottle hourly. This will ensure that you stay hydrated, maintain electrolytes, and receive the minimum in fuel. Take advantage of the aid stations along the way, but don't hang around more than five minutes. Stop just long enough to get fresh bottles, fill your pockets with food, and use the porta-johns. Lingering more than this may allow you to cool off and make it harder to get going again. Don't pig-out on the bike. This may not only cause nausea, but also divert blood from the muscles, where you need it most, to the gut for digestion.

If you trained properly and included adequate rest and tapering in the last week, the century should be no more difficult than your longest ride. In fact, it may even be easier because you're rested, nutritionally loaded, psyched up, and well-supported by volunteers.

Multiday Tours

On July 5, 1985, my family started a vacation we still talk about today. For 10 days we rode our bikes down the California coast from Crescent City in the north to San Diego in the south. We pedaled 880 miles unsupported. More importantly, we learned a lot about each other and created many memories, such as the day we ran out of food and water on Leggett Hill. We had started out that day with a planned stop for refueling in a small town on the map. It turned out to be a ghost town. We foraged through the woods and came up with a few handfuls of berries, enough fuel to get us to the next city a few hours down the road.

Then there was dodging the lumbering log trucks north of Fort Bragg, crossing *under* the Golden Gate Bridge on a catwalk due to construction, and suffering a flulike illness that struck in the last days of the trip—all trying adventures that became fond reminiscences.

Bike touring is unlike any other form of transportation. Instead of zipping along at 75 miles per hour in a car, on a bike you can truly see, smell, hear, and understand the countryside you travel through. People are friendlier and treat you differently than when you're in a car. Without even being asked, total strangers offer directions when you're lost, food when you're hungry, and even shelter when it rains. In addition, life is simpler when touring. No telephones, faxes, meetings, alarm clocks, or traffic jams. Each day is reduced to pedaling, eating, sleeping, and enjoying the companionship of friends. Seeing the world from the seat of a bike is an unbeatable experience.

If you're not ready for an unsupported tour, there are many companies and nonprofit fund-raisers providing two- to six-day road and off-road rides with lots of support. Amenities typical of such organized events are showers, meals, lodging, camping, sag wagons, bag transport, aid stations, mechanics, medical support, and massage. Your needs are well provided for; all you need do is turn the cranks.

It doesn't matter if you're a corporate CEO or an auto mechanic, once you're on a bike, everyone is the same. A bike helmet and shorts strip away the outward signs of status, allowing people to relax and get to know each other while facing a common challenge. You're all in this together. By day, all travel by the sweat of their own brows, and once in camp, celebrate and share the experience. The longer the tour, the deeper and longer lasting the newly formed friendships become.

Tour Training

The purpose of tour training is to develop enough endurance and resiliency to get back on the bike day after day. That's a lot different than getting fit for a single-day century ride, and the training is different, also. Preparing to tour places a greater emphasis on weekly mileage, or more specifically, time in the saddle, than does a century buildup in which weekly long rides were the dominant feature.

The century training schedules suggested in tables 5.2 and 5.4 rely on alternating hard and easy days of riding. This procedure ensures that the rider is fresh and rested before the critical workouts, many of which involve high intensity. Tour training, on the other hand, has little high intensity and the purpose is to get used to riding with accumulating fatigue while learning to quickly recover. Instead of separating the important rides with easy days, they are increasingly clumped together during the training buildup for a tour. This is called block training.

Block training is stressful, much more so than the hard-easy method. Because of this elevated stress, recovery weeks are only three weeks apart, instead of the more common four.

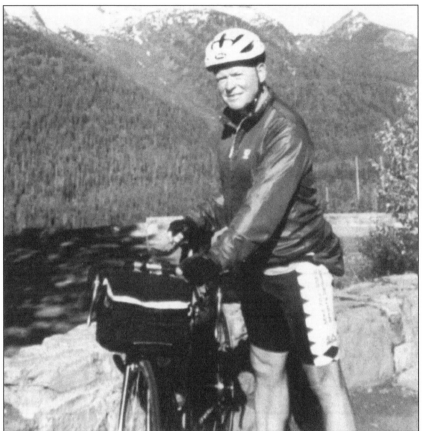

Going to Sun Highway. Glacier National Park, Montana.

You must also limit such training in terms of the number of continuous weeks you dedicate to it. Ten weeks is about the upper limit for most of us. This provides six weeks of block work, three rest and recovery weeks, and the tour start week.

Tables 5.6 and 5.7 provide suggested training routines for three-day and four- to six-day tours. Do the rides marked with * on courses similar to what you will ride on the tour for which you're preparing. If this will be hilly, you should be riding hills twice a week before even starting the 10-week buildup. If you will be riding the tour unsupported, do these marked rides with the loaded panniers you will use to get familiar with the changed steering, extra weight on the climbs, and downhill handling. Before starting either schedules, you should be

Table 5.6

TRAINING SCHEDULE FOR A THREE-DAY TOUR

Week	Mon	Tue	Wed	Thu	Fri	Sat	Sun	Total
10	Off	1:00	1:30*	Off	2:00*	1:00	3:00*	8:30
9	Off	1:00	1:00	1:30*	Off	3:00*	2:00*	8:30
8	Off	1:00	Off	1:00	Off	1:00	1:30*	4:30
7	Off	1:00	1:00	2:00*	Off	3:30*	2:00*	9:30
6	Off	1:00	1:00	2:00*	Off	3:30*	3:00*	10:30
5	Off	1:00	Off	1:00	Off	1:00	2:00*	5:00
4	Off	1:00	1:00	2:00*	Off	4:00*	3:00*	11:00
3	Off	1:00	1:00	Off	2:00*	4:30*	3:30*	12:00
2	Off	1:00	Off	1:00	Off	1:00	2:30*	5:30
1	Off	1:00	1:00	Off	Tour	Tour	Tour	2:00 + tour

*All times in hours:minutes; complete the rides marked * on terrain similar to the goal tour.

Table 5.7

TRAINING SCHEDULE FOR A FOUR- TO SIX-DAY TOUR

Week	Mon	Tue	Wed	Thu	Fri	Sat	Sun	Total
10	Off	1:00	1:00	1:30*	Off	3:00*	2:00*	8:30
9	Off	1:00	1:30	1:30*	Off	3:00*	2:00*	9:00
8	Off	1:00	Off	1:00	Off	1:00	2:00*	5:00
7	Off	1:00	1:30*	Off	2:00*	3:30*	2:00*	10:00
6	Off	1:00	1:30*	Off	2:00*	3:30*	2:30*	10:30
5	Off	1:00	Off	1:00	Off	1:00	2:30*	5:30
4	Off	1:00	1:30*	Off	2:30*	4:00*	3:00*	12:00
3	Off	1:00	Off	1:30*	2:30*	4:30*	3:30*	13:00
2	Off	1:00	Off	1:00*	Off	1:30	1:00	4:30
1	Off	1:00 or tour	Off or tour	Tour	Tour	Tour	Tour	1:00 + tour

*All times in hours:minutes; complete the rides marked * on terrain similar to the goal tour.

riding at least 8 hours per week, with a long ride of 2 hours 30 minutes or more.

Beyond Six Days

Tours that go beyond six days, such as cross-country riding, are unique. In one respect, getting the butt used to sitting on a saddle for several days, they are quite physically demanding. Yet the training and exertion level throughout is usually low key. If the distance to cover daily is less than 30 percent of your average weekly mileage in the previous six weeks before starting, and you're carrying all your gear on the bike, no special training is necessary. If you have a support vehicle carrying the gear, or you're credit-card touring instead of camping, you can probably handle 40 to 50 percent of your weekly mileage on any day. The exception to these guidelines would be if the tour will include several days of mountain climbing. In this case, lots of riding in the hills is necessary.

For a week or longer tour that frequently goes beyond your limits based on the previous guidelines, greater preparation is necessary. You'll have to get your weekly volume up by riding more frequently and with increasingly longer rides, using a pattern such as the one suggested in table 5.7. The key is to allow plenty of time to build your fitness and to increase your weekly volume by no more than 15 percent over the previous week's. Allowing every third week for rest and recovery will help to keep you from burning out before you start the tour.

Tour Tips

The intensity for all rides on tables 5.6 and 5.7, as in the tour itself, is primarily the heart rate 2 zone. On hills, allow the heart rate to rise to the 5a zone, but no higher. Shift to easier gears as the heart rate climbs to prevent going deeply anaerobic and accumulating lactate in the blood, which will cause fatigue. Learn to ride well within your limits on a daily basis to speed recovery for the following day. Staying with a pack of riders of similar ability will help you do this, as drafting at 20 miles per hour reduces the effort by about 25 percent. If possible, train with a group.

The position you assume when leading a group or riding alone determines how much energy you'll use. The racing position, with hands on the drops, requires about 15 percent less effort than riding in the upright position with hands on the bar tops. Aero bars further reduce effort.

Not only must your body be in shape, so must your bike. We recommend an overhaul of all moving parts before starting a multiday tour.

Racing

Racing is the ultimate test of a cyclist, whether it's a road race, mountain bike race, triathlon, or duathlon. Every race is an opportunity to challenge yourself as few other endeavors in our world offer. Races are intimidating, yet at the same time addictive.

Once over the initial fear of failure, which takes several starts, the new racer finds that past-50 competition is not as intimidating as imagined. Past-50 competitors race differently than the kids do. For one thing, they're less willing to take unnecessary risks. No race is worth a crash or injury. More importantly, there is a sense of community and support among the over-50 age group racers. They encourage novices and share training secrets. They accept each other, regardless of the results.

The feeling of kinship, however, doesn't lessen the desire of mature racers to perform to their utmost ability. Aging has not decreased the competitive spirit, only redefined it.

Those who think that past-50 means ready for the rocking chair have never gone for a ride with an aging bike racer. Many ride with cyclists younger than their children, yet give the youngsters all they can handle. The difference between the past-50 rider and his or her younger riding companions isn't so much in riding speed as it is in recovery. The older cyclists need more time between hard workouts and are more prone to injuries and overtraining. With more responsibilities, they also typically have less time to train than the 20-something cyclist. Fewer workouts mean less room for training mistakes.

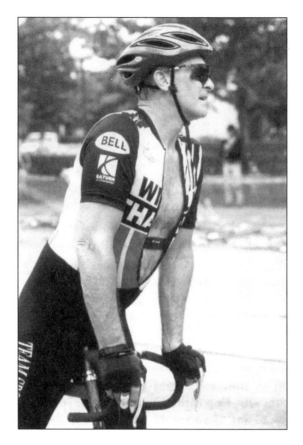

A race may be the mental challenge you are looking for.

Faced with this dilemma of getting more from less, the past-50 cyclist becomes wily. How to ride smarter, not harder, is the challenge. Planning is the solution.

Planning for the Perfect Peak

How did you come to the place in your business career that you are today? More than likely you didn't leave it to chance, but years ago decided what you needed in terms of education, skills, and experience to advance, and when you should gain these components of success. That's the way most successful business people get to the top. Yet, if you're like most racers, you've never considered planning a season so you come into top form at just the right times.

Over the years you've probably developed a method of training based on putting in a lot of miles in the late winter, then racing frequently in the spring. This race-into-shape system has been the standard in cycling for decades. Although you've undoubtedly produced some good results training this way, timing is a problem. Instead of being fit on race day, you're as likely to be flat. It's a crap shoot. There's no way to predict what will happen when races are months away and there's no definitive plan for peaking.

Besides the benefit of having predictable fitness at the right times, planned training is also time effective. When you schedule the components of fitness in advance, weekly workouts are routine and purposeful, just like a day at the office. You know what you need and you achieve it. No wasted time deciding what to do. No hit-or-miss decision making. You take the guesswork out of daily workouts, leaving you free to enjoy the ride. Getting on a bike knowing exactly what you have to do is a far different experience than rolling out of the driveway while trying to remember what you've recently done, how many days or weeks you have until your next important race, what your fitness needs are, and, finally, what you should do today. By the time you decide, you often discover you're going the wrong direction for the hills you need, or you wish you had a training partner to work on sprinting. Leaving training to chance is a sure way to waste a lot of time.

Preparing a plan is a confidence builder. Seeing the big picture by having a logical training progression on paper, and using it, provides a feeling of certainty about yourself and where you're going. In racing, we can all use a little more confidence.

There are three basic steps to take in planning a race season. This chapter will cover them all. They are, in the order of completion

1. goal setting,
2. annual planning, and
3. weekly workout planning.

Goals to Go the Distance

Let's start at the beginning. The way to race more successfully is to know exactly what you want from racing. Not having race goals is like starting a car trip without a destination in mind. You'll certainly wind up somewhere, but perhaps not where you'd like to be.

Although you've probably followed a goal-setting procedure like the one described here in other endeavors, you may not have applied it to cycling. Following these seven goal-setting steps will put you ahead of the competition before turning the cranks the first time.

Own the Goal

Before deciding what the first goal is, realize that for success, the goal must be your own. It can't be something your spouse or friend thinks you should or could accomplish. If there isn't a burning personal desire to achieve a goal, it will wither and die. Disregard what others want. What is it *you* want from racing?

Believe the Goal

Believable goals are the ones you will work toward. If you're new to racing, winning a national championship is only a remote possibility, and one you'd realize down deep is not worth the effort. Finishing your first race is a believable and realistic goal. Although the goal must stretch you, it can't be so far beyond your ability to achieve, given the time and talents you have, that you are unmotivated by it. What you truly believe, you can achieve.

Write the Goal

Writing your goals is a powerful incentive. The physical act of recording goals burns them into your consciousness and helps make them believable. A good place to record goals is on a place marker in your training diary where you can see them every time you open it. What you write down should be performance oriented, not turnstile goals. An example of a performance goal is, "Break one hour for 40-kilometer time trial." A turnstile goal is, "Attend six races." Turnstile goals are not as likely to stretch your limits as performance goals are.

Measure the Goal

Decide what the fitness limiters (endurance, climbing, sprinting, time trialing) are in achieving each goal, and determine where you presently stand on each. For example, you may need the ability to ride two hours in the heart rate 3 zone, or time trial 20 kilometers at an average speed of 23 miles per hour, or sprint 200 meters at an average power of 500 watts. How do you stack up against these standards now? How will you know when you're ready? Here's a simple way of answering these questions. If in training you can achieve the goal's full *quality* (3 zone, 20 miles per hour, 500 watts) for half of the goal's stated *quantity* (two hours, 20 kilometers, 200 meters), you can probably achieve the entire goal's quality and quantity in a race. This makes it easy to set short-term and measurable supporting objectives for a goal. For example, if you want to complete a 20-kilometer time trial at 23 miles per hour, the objective for such a goal could be, "Ride 10 kilometers at an average speed of 23 miles per hour two weeks before XYZ race." You now have something to aim at in workouts.

Time the Goal

Setting deadlines for performance goals is easy. All you need to know is when the races are. The tricky part is setting deadlines for the supporting objectives along the way. It's usually best to allow a little more time than you think is necessary. The example in the previous step did this by allowing for attainment of the supporting objective two weeks before the race. Targeting these objective deadlines on your daily calendar will keep you focused.

Support the Goal

Decide who you need to help achieve your goals. This may be teammates, friends, or spouse. Anyone who can lend you moral or physical help along the way needs to know what your most important goals are. Don't tell others, especially those who are negative and always finding what's wrong in life. These people will only hold you back. The best way to get support for your goals is to support the goals of others.

Plan the Goal

A goal without a plan is a wish. Deciding exactly what to accomplish, by when, and writing it down provides a road map for the trip. Just as when traveling, you may decide to make some changes along the way, so write in pencil or put it on a computer to make adjustments easy. The next section leads you through a systematic and concise planning method.

Annual Planning Pointers

Now that you've set the season's goals, you can design a plan that will achieve them. Without goals, planning is an empty task that merely organizes the use of time. With goals, planning becomes a tool for achieving them, and for developing fitness logically and effectively. The plan you will develop here is based on the concept of periodization described in chapter 3. There are six steps in the planning process. For reference as you go through the steps, table 6.1 illustrates a typical annual training plan for a race season.

Table 6.1

ANNUAL TRAINING PLAN FOR A TWO-PEAK SEASON WITH 10 WEEKS BETWEEN PEAKS

Weeks	Races	Periods	Hours
1		Prep	8.5
2		Prep	8.5
3		Prep	8.5
4		Prep	8.5
5		Base 1	10.0
6		Base 1	12.0
7		Base 1	13.5
8		Base 1	7.0
9		Base 2	10.5
10		Base 2	12.5
11		Base 2	14.0
12		Base 2	7.0
13		Base 3	11.0
14		Base 3	13.5
15		Base 3	15.0
16		Base 3	7.0
17		Build 1	12.5
18		Build 1	12.5
19	C race	Build 1	7.0
20		Build 2	12.0
21		Build 2	12.0
22	C race	Build 2	7.0
23		Build 3	12.0

(continued)

(continued)

Weeks	Races	Periods	Hours
24		Build 3	12.0
25	C race	Build 3	7.0
26	C race	Peak	10.5
27	B race	Peak	8.5
28	A race	Race	7.0
29	B race	Race	7.0
30	A race	Race	7.0
31		Transition	7.0
32		Base 3	13.5
33		Base 3	15.0
34	C race	Base 3	7.0
35	C race	Build 2	12.0
36		Build 2	12.0
37	B race	Build 2	7.0
38	C race	Build 3	12.0
39		Build 3	12.0
40	B race	Build 3	7.0
41	B race	Peak	10.5
42	B race	Peak	8.5
43	A race	Race	7.0
44	B race	Race	7.0
45	A race	Race	7.0
46	B race	Race	7.0
47		Transition	7.0
48		Transition	7.0
49		Transition	7.0
50		Transition	7.0
51		Prep	8.5
52		Prep	8.5

Based on 500 annual training hours

Step 1. Decide Race Priorities

Make a list of all the races you may do during the season. If in doubt about any, include them in the list. Next, decide how important each is using the following criteria.

A-priority races are the most important on your schedule. They are critical to your season goals. There should be only two to four of them. The exception is when there are two A races in the same week or a stage race; count this as one A race. You

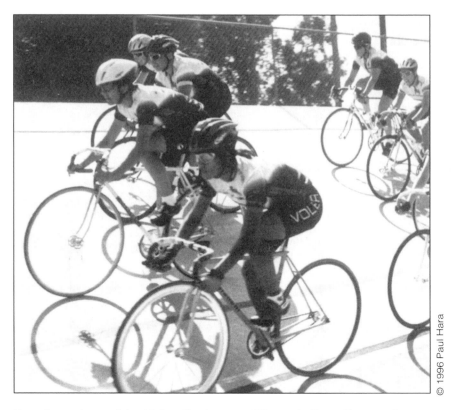

© 1996 Paul Hara

Tara Spangler and the Valley Spokesmen Women's Race Team train at the Hellyer Park Velodrome in San Jose, California.

will design your season around these events, building to a fitness peak and tapering before them. If you designate four A races, at least two of them should be clumped into a two- to four-week period for best results. Spreading four out with six or more weeks separation makes it difficult to rebuild fitness and peak for each one.

B-priority races are important and you want to do well at them, but they are not as important to your season's goals as the A races. You will rest for a few days before these, but not peak and taper. There may be up to eight B-priority races in a season.

C-priority races are the least important ones on the schedule and are there as tune-ups before A and B races, and for experience, fun, or because others, such as teammates, want you to do them. There may be doubt right up to the last few days before a C race about whether you'll do it. The race outcome is not tied to your goals, so you will train through these, using them as hard workouts only. Be careful how many of these you do, as they can leave you too tired to train for several days. Riders with several years of racing experience and challenging season goals should be especially wary of C races, as there is little to be gained and high potential for setback.

Step 2. Schedule Peak and Race Periods

On a calendar, using a pencil, or on computer calendar software, write in all the races you listed, along with their A, B, or C designations, on the appropriate days. Count two weeks backward from each A-priority race or the first A race in a two- to four-week clump. Designate this two-week period as a Peak period on the calendar. It's best to have no more than three, and preferably only two, Peak periods in your schedule with a wide separation of six or more weeks between them. Follow each Peak period by a Race period that includes one, two, or three A-priority races and perhaps some B-priority races in a one- to four-week period. Later in this chapter you will learn what the Peak and Race periods, and the other periods to follow, mean for training.

Step 3. Schedule Build Periods

Designate the three weeks before each two-week peak period as Build 3, the three weeks before that as Build 2, and the next three weeks as Build 1. You will develop race-specific fitness in these periods with the last week of each Build period as a rest and recovery week. These R and R weeks are critical to your success, and you should never leave them out. During an R and R week, greatly reduce training volume as you rest, and at the end of the week you should have a test of progress or a race.

If there are less than six weeks between the end of a Race period and the start of the next Peak period, and the previous Race period was two weeks or less, include only Build 2 and Build 3. Keep Build 3 at three weeks, and reduce Build 2 to fit the time frame. For example, if there are only five weeks between A races and the preceding Race period was two weeks long, keep Build 3 as three weeks and assign two weeks to Build 2 before starting the next Peak period.

If the previous Race period was three or four weeks long and there are less than six weeks until the next Peak, return to Build 1 and 2. Keep Build 1 as three weeks and reduce Build 2 to fit the calendar. The reason is that the longer the Race period, the more endurance you potentially lose. Build 1 offers more endurance training than the later Build periods.

If there are more than six weeks between Race and Peak periods, assign six weeks to a Build 2-Build 3 combination. The first week after the Race period is a Transition period (more on this later), and the remaining weeks are Base 3.

Step 4. Schedule Base Periods

The weeks before your first Build 1 are designated as a Base 3 period, which will now be four weeks long instead of the three we've been using. In the same manner, assign a four-week Base 2 and, still working backward, a four-week Base 1. During the Base periods develop endurance, strength, and pedaling skills. These periods are longer as they aren't as stressful as the Build periods and require less frequent rest and recovery.

For a multipeak season with A races separated by more than 12 weeks, it's generally a good idea to schedule another Base 3 period following the first Race period. This will reestablish the basic elements of fitness, helping to make the next Peak a higher one.

Step 5. Schedule Transition and Prep Periods

At the end of your last Race period of the season, assign two to four weeks for Transition. This is a period of reduced training with little or no regimentation. It's a time to fully recover from the previous season's increasing tedium of training and racing by doing things other than riding a bike. During the racing year, whenever there are more than six weeks between the end of a Race period and the next Peak period, schedule a transition week immediately following the Race period. This will keep you mentally sharp and highly motivated to train.

The Prep period is a time to regain cardiorespiratory fitness following a three- or four-week Transition. It can be two to eight weeks long and precedes the next season's Base 1.

Step 6. Assign Weekly Hours

The number of hours you train each week has an impact on race performance. Too few and you are undertrained for longer events. Too many and the risk of overtraining rises. The starting point for assigning weekly volume is to determine the number of hours of training for the year. One way to do this is to total your training hours for the previous 12 months. If you don't keep track of hours, but record miles, divide that total by an estimate of average speed. So, if you rode 4,250 miles with assumed average speed of 16 miles per hour, your estimate of annual hours on the bike is 265 (4,250 ÷ 16 = 265.6). If you keep track of neither hours or miles, take an educated guess. Also, add any cross-training hours, such as productive time in the weight room, running, cross-country skiing, and aerobics classes. Annual training hours include all physical activities within a year that may have a direct benefit for racing fitness.

Table 6.2 suggests typical annual training hours for past-50 riders by sport and race level. It's possible that your annual hours are well below those of the race level at which you aspire or currently perform. You may even put in more hours than suggested, but fail to achieve the performance standards on this table. This takes us back to the principle of individualization described in chapter 3. When it comes to training, each of us is an experiment with one subject. If you decide to increase your annual training hours, do so conservatively. A 15 percent change is a lot.

Knowing annual training hours allows you to now assign weekly training hours using table 6.3. Find your annual hours column for each training period, and write the weekly hours

Table 6.2

TYPICAL PAST-50 ANNUAL TRAINING HOURS

Race level	Road racing	Mountain bike	Triathlon
Finisher	200-300	200-300	300-400
Midpack	300-400	300-400	400-500
Competitive	400-600	400-500	500-600
National class	500-700	500-600	600-700

Table 6.3

WEEKLY TRAINING HOURS BY PERIOD

Period	Week	200	250	300	350	400	450	500	550	600	650	700
Prep	All	4.0	4.0	5.0	6.0	7.0	7.5	8.5	9.0	10.0	11.0	12.0
Base 1	1	4.0	5.0	6.0	7.0	8.0	9.0	10.0	11.0	12.0	12.5	14.0
	2	5.0	6.0	7.0	8.5	9.5	10.5	12.0	13.0	14.5	15.5	16.5
	3	5.5	6.5	8.0	9.5	10.5	12.0	13.5	14.5	16.0	17.5	18.5
	4	4.0	4.0	4.0	5.0	5.5	6.5	7.0	8.0	8.5	9.0	10.0
Base 2	1	4.0	5.5	6.5	7.5	8.5	9.5	10.5	12.5	12.5	13.0	14.5
	2	5.0	6.5	7.5	9.0	10.0	11.5	12.5	14.0	15.0	16.5	17.5
	3	5.5	7.0	8.5	10.0	11.0	12.5	14.0	15.5	17.0	18.0	19.5
	4	4.0	4.0	4.5	5.0	5.5	6.5	7.0	8.0	8.5	9.0	10.0
Base 3	1	4.5	5.5	7.0	8.0	9.0	10.0	11.0	12.5	13.5	14.5	15.5
	2	5.0	6.5	8.0	9.5	10.5	12.0	13.5	14.5	16.0	17.0	18.5
	3	6.0	7.5	9.0	10.5	11.5	13.0	15.0	16.5	18.0	19.0	20.5
	4	4.0	4.0	4.5	5.0	5.5	6.5	7.0	8.0	8.5	9.0	10.0
Build 1	1	5.0	6.5	8.0	9.0	10.0	11.5	12.5	14.0	15.5	16.0	17.5
	2	5.0	6.5	8.0	9.0	10.0	11.5	12.5	14.0	15.5	16.0	17.5
	3	4.0	4.0	4.5	5.0	5.5	6.5	7.0	8.0	8.5	9.0	10.0
Build 2	1	5.0	6.0	7.0	8.5	9.5	10.5	12.0	13.0	14.5	15.5	16.5
	2	5.0	6.0	7.0	8.5	9.5	10.5	12.0	13.0	14.5	15.5	16.5
	3	4.0	4.0	4.5	5.0	5.5	6.5	7.0	8.0	8.5	9.0	10.0
Build 3	1	5.0	6.0	7.0	8.5	9.5	10.5	12.0	13.0	14.5	15.5	16.5
	2	5.0	6.0	7.0	8.5	9.5	10.5	12.0	13.0	14.5	15.5	16.5
	3	4.0	4.0	4.5	5.0	5.5	6.5	7.0	8.0	8.0	8.5	10.0
Peak	1	5.0	5.5	6.5	7.5	8.5	9.5	10.5	11.5	13.0	13.5	14.5
	2	4.0	5.0	5.0	6.0	6.5	7.5	8.5	9.5	10.0	11.0	11.5
Race	All	4.0	4.0	4.5	5.0	5.5	6.5	7.0	8.0	8.5	9.0	10.0
Transition	All	4.0	4.0	4.5	5.0	5.5	6.5	7.0	8.0	8.5	9.0	10.0

from the chart at the start of each week on the calendar. The longest ride in most weeks should be at least as long as your longest race. Divide the other workouts, including weights and cross-training, between the remaining hours. Races, weightlifting, and cross-training all count as training hours. These weekly hours are merely a guide. Don't think of them as an absolute standard that you must meet under all circumstances. It's likely you'll have to make frequent changes in them as circumstances dictate.

Weekly Workouts

Once you have a periodization plan for the season, it's time to look at the specifics of weekly training. How to train on a daily basis varies between sports for most periods of the year. Some periods, however, are the same regardless of sport. The Transition, Prep, and Base periods follow similar training patterns for road racing, mountain biking, triathlon, and duathlon.

The following description of each training period discusses only the bike portion of training. Triathletes and duathletes will also need to blend swimming and running into each period. You may do this by emphasizing the bike one week and running the next, while swimming remains a constant. Another way is to put slightly more emphasis on the weaker sport, cycling or running, each week and keeping swimming the same. Table 6.4 provides a list of workouts to choose from in designing each week's training rides. It also suggests the best periods to use these workouts.

Transition Period

The purpose of this period is to recover, mentally and physically, from the stresses of high-level training. In the plan just completed, you probably scheduled two of these periods, one early in the race season following the first Race period and another following the last race period. Without breaks from training such as these, the possibility of burnout is high in motivated riders. Taking a break permits starting into hard training again with a renewed enthusiasm.

Table 6.4

WORKOUT MENU

WORKOUT	DESCRIPTION	INTENSITY	CADENCE	PERIOD
Cardiorespiratory endurance—Improve heart and lung function				
Cross-training	Run, swim, ski, etc.	Low to moderate	N/A	Transition
Aerobic Endurance—Improve ability to deliver and use oxygen				
Recovery ride	Flat course, trainer	HR 1	84-100	All
Long, slow distance	Ride mostly flat	HR 1-2	84-100	All
Endurance brick	Long bike + run	HR 1-3	84-100	Build 1, Build 2
Strength—Increase force applied to pedals				
Rolling hills	Seated	HR 1-4	50+	All
Moderate, long hills	Seated	HR 1-5a	50+	Base 2 and all following
Steep, short hills	Sit or stand	HR 1-5b	50+	Build 1 and all following
Weights	See chapter 8	Varies	N/A	All except Transition
Leg speed—Develop ability to turn pedals at high cadence				
Spin-ups	Repeat max spins	N/A	120+	Prep, Base 1, Base 2
Isolated leg training	1-leg pedaling	N/A	80+	Prep, Base 1, Base 2
Form sprints	Tailwind sprints	N/A	120+	Base 3, Build 1
Fixed gear	Flat to rolling	HR 1-3	90+	Base 1, Base 2
Sprints	8-12" (3-5')	N/A	120+	Build 1 and following
Skills—Improve event-specific handling skills				
Bumping	On grass with partner	N/A	N/A	Base 1, Base 2, Base 3
Cornering	No traffic area	N/A	N/A	Base 1, Base 2, Base 3
Pace lines	Group ride	N/A	N/A	Base 1, Base 2, Base 3
Balancing	Track stands, hops	N/A	N/A	Base 1, Base 2, Base 3

MTB technical	Challenging terrain	N/A	N/A	Base 3 and following
Aero position	Bike adjustments	N/A	N/A	Base 1, Base 2, Base 3

Muscular endurance—Improve lactate threshold speed, endurance, and comfort

Tempo	20'+ continuous	HR 3	90+	Base 2, Base 3
Cruise intervals	3-5 × 6-12' (2-3')	HR 4-5a	84+	Base 3 and all following
Hill cruise intervals	2-4% grade	HR 4-5a	60+	Base 3 and all following
MTB hill cruise intervals	Shift up-down @ 30"	HR 4-5a	50-90	Build 2, Build 3, Peak
Threshold	20'+ continuous	HR 4-5a	84+	Build 2, Build 3, Peak
Crisscross threshold	Vary HR high to low	HR 4-5a	84+	Build 2, Build 3, Peak
Race-tempo brick	Half race distance	Race effort	84+	Build 3 and following

Speed endurance—Improve aerobic capacity, lactate tolerance, long sprints

SE intervals	3-5 × 3-6' (3-6')	HR 5b	90+	Build 1 and following
Hill SE intervals	6-8% grade	HR 5b	60+	Build 2 and following
Pyramid intervals	1-2-3-4-4-3-2-1'	HR 5b	90+	Build 2 and following
Lactate tolerance reps	4-8 × 1.5-2' (4-5')	HR 5c	100+	Build 3 Peak
MTB starts	5' max, 10' t-hold	Max, HR 4-5a	Increase	Build 2 and following

Anaerobic power—Improve instantaneous force application to pedals

Jumps	10-25 × 10-12 rpm	Max effort	To max	Base 3 and following
Hill sprints	6-9 × 20" (5'), 4%	Max effort	70-80	Build 1 and following
Crit sprints	6-9 × 30" (5'), turns	Max effort	Varies	Build 2 and following
Match sprints	6-9 × 20" (5')	Max effort	Varies	Peak, Race

Special workouts

Warm-up	Practice warm-up	Varies	Varies	Build 1 and following
Race simulation	Group ride	Race effort	Varies	Build 1 and following
MTB starts	5' max, 10' threshold	Race effort	Varies	Build 3, Peak

*Minutes are indicated as ' and seconds as "; times in parentheses are recovery intervals.

During the Transition period, the only guidelines are (1) cut way back on volume and intensity, (2) stay active doing something besides riding the bike, and (3) have fun. Other than occasional rides and cross-training, make up for time lost during the season with your family.

Prep Period

The Prep period is a time of training to train. During this period the focus is cardiorespiratory fitness and preparing the muscles and tendons for heavier strength training as training volume increases slightly. You can use the bike as a primary mode of training at this time, but in the northern states that may not be possible, other than on an indoor trainer, due to winter weather. Any aerobic activity done at moderate intensity will improve cardiorespiratory fitness. The possibilities are many, including swimming, cross-country skiing, running, rowing, hiking, aerobics classes, and stair-climbing machines. If you can't ride outside due to short days, cold temperatures, or snow, using an indoor trainer, such as rollers, a wind load or magnetic trainer, CompuTrainer, or Cycle Ops Electronic Trainer is acceptable, but don't overdo it as there is plenty of that in the Base period coming up next. Cross-training is preferable to extensive indoor riding at this time.

A typical weekly training pattern in the Prep period includes two or three days of strength training separated by 48 to 72 hours, three or four aerobic workouts in the heart rate 1 or 2 zones, and a day off. The Anatomical Adaptation strength training phase for the Prep period is described in chapter 8.

Base 1 Period

Training starts in earnest in the Base 1 period, increasing weekly hours as shown in table 6.3 and gradually stepping up intensity. By the end of this four-week period you should have developed greater aerobic endurance and strength, and improved pedaling skills. Do pedaling drills annually, regardless of how many years you've been riding. They're the basics, the fundamentals of bicycle pedaling. They're described under Sprint Workouts in chapter 4 as *Spin-ups* and *Isolated leg*.

Each of the first three weeks of Base 1 typically includes a workout of at least 90 minutes in the heart rate 1 or 2 zones, two weight sessions, one or two leg-speed workouts, one or two aerobic workouts in the 1 to 3 zones on the bike or other mode, and a day off. The weight-room strength phase is called maximum strength (MS) (see chapter 8). Table 6.5 suggests a typical week in Base 1.

During all three Base periods you do in the winter months, an indoor trainer may be the only option for getting time on the bike in the northern states. Limit these to 90 minutes, tops. Whenever you must ride inside for the third consecutive day, do some other aerobic exercise such as those listed in the Prep period. Many long hours on an indoor trainer can lead to a loss of enthusiasm for cycling. Enthusiasm is always preferable to fitness.

In the fourth week, the R and R week, cut the long workout by a third, do half as many sets of weights in each workout, and reduce training time of the other workouts. This is a good time to establish a baseline of your aerobic fitness with the aerobic time trial described in chapter 3. The R and R week is the same in each of the Base periods.

Base 2 Period

In the second Base period, start weekly volume a little higher than where Base 1 began (table 6.3), and finish it three weeks later at a yet higher level. Introduce two new elements of training, slightly increasing the intensity of training. The first is strength work in the hills. The moderate hill workout described in chapter 4 will begin converting the maximum

Table 6.5

TYPICAL BASE 1 TRAINING WEEK

Monday	Weights (MS phase)
Tuesday	Pedaling skills
Wednesday	Aerobic training
Thursday	Weights (MS phase)
Friday	Day off
Saturday	Aerobic training or pedaling skills
Sunday	Long, aerobic ride

strength gains made in the weight room in Base 1 into better climbing strength. The other new training element is muscular endurance (ME). Do the tempo workout from chapter 4, with extended rides on flat courses and heart rate in the 3 zone, once a week, including the R and R week. Weight work moves into the power endurance (PE) phase as you convert raw strength to a more useable form for cycling.

In addition to the weekly hill ride, tempo workout, and two weight-room sessions, there should be one day of leg-speed drills and a long, aerobic-endurance ride. For road racers new to the sport, you may alternate the pedaling drills day with a day of working on skills. You can use a parking lot or low-traffic neighborhood to practice high-speed cornering, using different combinations of leaning the bike or the body and approach angles. Novice mountain bikers may also work on balancing technical handling skills. The long ride is now at least two hours to further develop aerobic endurance. As always, take one day off from training weekly. Table 6.6 shows how you can arrange a Base 2 week.

Base 3 Period

This is the final period of general fitness development. By the end of this period, you must be ready to begin training at race intensities. To prepare for that, increase volume to the highest level of the season and raise intensity a bit. Weight training is less demanding now, and you should use cross-training only when the weather forces it, as you reserve more energy for riding. This is the last big push before reducing volume and

Table 6.6

TYPICAL BASE 2 TRAINING WEEK	
Monday	Weights (PE phase)
Tuesday	Pedaling skills
Wednesday	Hill training
Thursday	Weights (PE phase)
Friday	Day off
Saturday	Tempo ride
Sunday	Long, aerobic ride

dramatically increasing intensity in the Build 1 period and possible start of C-priority races.

The first three weeks of Base 3 include five types of workouts, all extensions of what you did before. Table 6.7 shows how you can schedule these workouts.

The long ride is still a staple of training. Such rides now become the longest of the season, going beyond the anticipated duration of the longest race on the schedule. You can do these on moderate hills, especially for those whose limiter, as discovered in chapter 4, is climbing. Heart rate is mostly in the 1 to 3 zones, with some 4 and 5a zones only when climbing.

Also include one shorter hill ride each week, now on long hills as described in chapter 4. Climb these hills staying in the saddle with the cadence at least at 50 revolutions per minute. Should your knees feel tender, use a lower gear with a higher cadence, climb standing more often, or skip the hills altogether. No amount of fitness is worth an injury.

The muscular endurance work you began in Base 2 now shifts from tempo rides in the heart rate 3 zone to cruise intervals in the 4 and 5a zones. These are especially beneficial for riders with a limiter in time trialing. If the limiter is climbing, you can do these on a hill with a moderate grade up to 4 percent. Triathletes should do this workout on a bike set up with aero bars. Cruise intervals are explained in chapter 4.

Skills training from the previous Base periods now becomes more race specific. Once a week, road racers should do form sprints, occasionally including cornering; mountain bikers work on handling skills off road; and triathletes practice riding in the aero position with a slightly higher-than-normal

Table 6.7

TYPICAL BASE 3 TRAINING WEEK

Monday	Weights (ME phase)
Tuesday	Skills training
Wednesday	Hills training
Thursday	Weights (ME phase)
Friday	Day off
Saturday	Cruise intervals
Sunday	Long, aerobic ride

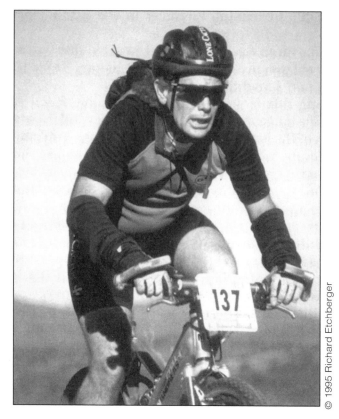

© 1995 Richard Etchberger

Mountain bike races can be described as "a time trial starting with a sprint."

cadence. A mountain biker whose handling skills need work may now want to do the Wednesday hill ride off road.

Weight training is less demanding in this period. Do the muscular endurance phase twice weekly. If you have the time, it's a good idea to spin at a comfortably high cadence on a trainer or rollers for 20 to 30 minutes later the same day as a weight workout. This will give you more training time while reminding your muscles how to make quick, smooth circles.

Coming Into Race Form

At the conclusion of the Base periods, the basic fitness elements of cardiorespiratory and aerobic endurance, strength from weight and hill training, and leg speed should be quite high. Muscular endurance should be coming along, too. In the following periods, Build, Peak, and Race, the intensity of training increases as workouts become more racelike. Table 6.8 shows this gradual shift away from aerobic volume and climbing to intervals and time-trial workouts.

For the first time in the young season, training shifts from emphasizing volume with increasingly longer rides and greater weekly hours, to emphasizing intensity with decreasing volume. If the Base periods have gone well, there will be little difficulty maintaining aerobic fitness with a weekly long ride of at least race duration. The B- and C-priority races that you may introduce in the Build and Peak periods also serve as high-intensity workouts. During these race weeks, replace the highest intensity workouts with low-intensity rides. Figure 6.1 summarizes the changes that now occur in the relative mix of volume and intensity.

On weekends in the Build and Peak periods, when there is a short race such as a criterium or sprint-distance triathlon, it may be necessary to ride for an hour or more after the race to cool down and maintain aerobic base. Longer races, of course, will not require such a long add-on, but may still include a cooldown ride.

Build 1 Period

In the Build 1 period, the gradual change to higher intensity comes by introducing speed-endurance (SE) intervals as discussed in chapter 4. These are especially important for the criterium racer, for whom intermittent high speeds closely simulate the event, and slightly less so for the road racer, mountain biker, triathlete, and duathlete. A weekly session at the introductory level of this workout will bring aerobic fitness to a peak at the right time. For each of the first two weeks of Build 1, do a workout such as four times three minutes, building to the heart rate 5b zone with three-minute recoveries, 4 × 3 minutes @ 5b (3 minutes @ 1). The three-minute work interval begins as soon as you increase force on the pedals, *not* when you achieve the 5b zone. In the next week, add one work interval to make it 5 × 3 minutes @ 5b (3 minutes @ 1). Complete this workout on a flat stretch of road with low traffic.

Table 6.8

PERIODIZATION OF TRAINING BY WORKOUT TYPE

Workout type	Prep	Base 1	Base 2	Base 3	Build 1	Build 2	Build 3	Peak	Race	Transition
Endurance— Cardiorespiratory	2									1
Endurance— Aerobic (volume)	1	3	4	5	3	2	2	1	1	
Endurance— Aerobic (intervals)					1	2	3	2		
Endurance— Muscular/ Time Trial		1	2	3	4	3	3	2	1	
Climb		1	3	4	3	3	2	1		
Skills, sprinting		1	1	2	2	2	2	3	2	
Strength—AA	4									
Strength—MS		3								
Strength—PE			3		1		1			
Strength—ME				2		1		1		

1 = low emphasis; 2 = low-moderate emphasis; 3 = moderate emphasis; 4 = moderate-high emphasis; 5 = high emphasis

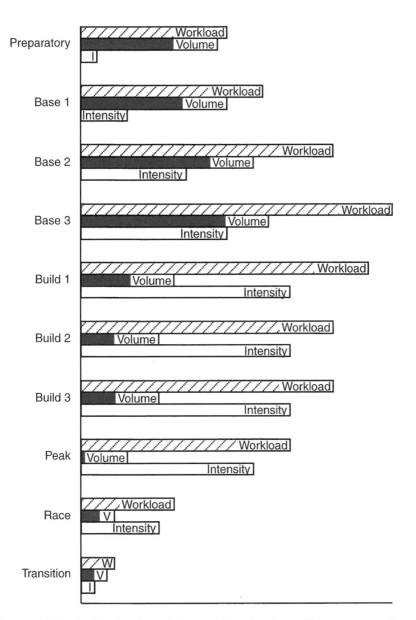

Figure 6.1 Periodization by relative workload, volume (frequency and time), and intensity

Road racers may include three to five sprints in the warm-up before the intervals begin.

Mountain bikers and triathletes should do this workout alone. Road racers may do it with another rider, alternating pulls every three minutes to more closely simulate race conditions. If, however, your heart rate won't drop into the 2 zone or lower while in the draft position, you're better off alone. Otherwise, the workout will become overly stressful, requiring greater recovery time.

Triathletes and duathletes are also increasing the intensity of running workouts in Build 1. Heart rate training zones for running are about 5 to 10 beats per minute higher than cycling zones. In lieu of completing a test on a treadmill, similar to the lactate threshold heart rate test described in chapter 4 to discover running zones, try adding seven beats to each cycling zone. This should be close and will work until you can complete such a test for running.

The other significant change to make in the Build 1 period is introducing race-specific workouts. Road racers, for example, should start doing group rides, especially on hilly terrain. These rides become increasingly racelike as the three Build periods progress. Mountain bikers should do a trail ride on a hilly route, increasing the intensity weekly until the workouts become much like races. A companion of similar ability is beneficial for these rides. To train race specificity, triathletes and duathletes may begin endurance bricks by combining a bike ride with a run. The total duration of this workout should be between 90 minutes and 2 and 1/2 hours for races up to international distance, and as much as 5 hours for an Ironman-distance race. In addition, the multisport athlete should include a hilly ride weekly.

Otherwise, training in Build 1 remains similar to Base 3, with cruise intervals now becoming somewhat longer as you reduce weight training, power endurance (PE) phase, to one day per week. Table 6.9 provides a suggested weekly routine for the Build 1 period.

Build 2 Period

In Build 2, the biggest change is progressing from cruise intervals to threshold workouts for developing muscular endurance. Threshold rides are controlled time trials with the

Table 6.9

TYPICAL BUILD 1 TRAINING WEEK

	Road racer	Mountain biker	Triathlete
Monday	Weights (ME phase)	Weights (ME phase)	Weights (ME phase) + swim
Tuesday	Cruise intervals	Cruise intervals	Run cruise intervals
Wednesday	Recovery ride or off	Recovery road ride or off	Recovery ride + swim
Thursday	Aerobic capacity (AC) intervals	AC intervals	Run + bike AC intervals
Friday	Day off	Day off	Day off or swim
Saturday	Group ride in hills	Hilly trail ride	Endurance brick
Sunday	Long, aerobic ride	Long, aerobic road ride	Bike in hills

Table 6.10

TYPICAL BUILD 2 TRAINING WEEK

	Road racer	Mountain biker	Triathlete
Monday	Weights (SM phase)	Weights (SM phase)	Weights (SM phase) + swim
Tuesday	Threshold ride	Threshold ride	Run cruise intervals
Wednesday	Recovery ride or off	Recovery road ride or off	Recovery ride + swim
Thursday	Aerobic capacity intervals	AC intervals on hill	Run + bike AC intervals
Friday	Day off	Day off	Day off or swim
Saturday	Group ride in hills	Hilly trail ride	Endurance brick
Sunday	Long, aerobic ride	Long, aerobic road ride	Bike in hills

heart rate in the 4 and 5a zones. These are best done alone on a flat course with no stops and light traffic.

Road racers and multisport athletes now extend the duration of SE intervals. This could be, for example, 4 × 4 minutes @ 5b (4 minutes @ 1) the first week, and 4 × 5 minutes @ 5b (5 minutes @ 1) the second. Because power climbs are typical of off-road racing, mountain bikers may now move their intervals to a moderately steep, off-road hill of 6- to 8-percent grade and do workouts such as 4 × 4 minutes @ 5b (4 minutes @ 1) and 5 × 4 minutes @ 5b (4 minutes @ 1).

The only other change in Build 2 is the muscular endurance (ME) phase of strength training, replacing the power endurance phase for the single weekly session in the weight room. Otherwise, training remains similar to Build 1 as shown in table 6.10.

Build 3 Period

This period is a continuation of Build 2 with only small modifications. The first is to lengthen the threshold workouts to 30- or 40-minute continuous efforts. Another is that road racers and multisport athletes move their SE intervals to hills, doing the same workouts the mountain bikers did in Build 2, except on paved roads. Mountain bikers may seek a steeper (greater than 8-percent grade) and shorter hill for these intervals and do something such as 4 × 3 minutes @ 5b (3 minutes @ 1), followed the next week by 5 × 3 minutes @ 5b (3 minutes @ 1). Everything else in the training week remains the same for road racers and mountain bikers.

Triathletes and duathletes may substitute race-tempo bricks for endurance bricks. These involve a bike-run workout at half the distance of the target race at race pace. The ability to hold race pace for half the race distance in a workout is a good indicator of race readiness. You can now drop the hilly bike workout of previous periods in favor of a flatter course ridden in the heart rate 1 and 2 zones. Table 6.11 illustrates a typical Build 3 training pattern for all three sports.

Build Period R and R Weeks

As with all previous training periods, the last week is always for R and R. In the Build periods this happens every third week,

Table 6.11

TYPICAL BUILD 3 TRAINING WEEK

	Road racer	Mountain biker	Triathlete
Monday	Weights (SM phase)	Weights (SM phase)	Weights (SM phase) + swim
Tuesday	Threshold ride	Threshold ride	Run cruise intervals
Wednesday	Recovery ride or off	Recovery road ride or off	Recovery ride + swim
Thursday	AC intervals on hill	AC intervals on hill	Run + bike AC intervals on hill
Friday	Day off	Day off	Day off or swim
Saturday	Group ride in hills	Hilly trail ride	Tempo brick
Sunday	Long, aerobic ride	Long, aerobic road ride	Long, aerobic ride

Table 6.12

TYPICAL BUILD R AND R WEEK

	Road racer	Mountain biker	Triathlete
Monday	Weights (50% sets)	Weights (50% sets)	Weights (50% sets) + swim
Tuesday	Recovery ride or off	Recovery ride or off	Day off
Wednesday	Cruise intervals	Cruise intervals	Run cruise intervals
Thursday	Recovery ride	Recovery ride	Recovery ride
Friday	Day off	Day off	Swim
Saturday	Group ride or race	Hilly trail ride or race	Tempo brick or race
Sunday	Recovery ride or off	Recovery ride or off	Recovery ride or off

instead of every fourth as in the Base periods. There are three purposes for R and R weeks during the Build period. The first, and most important, is to allow rest and recovery from the previous two weeks. The second is to maintain muscular endurance by including shortened cruise intervals. The third is to gauge progress by finishing the week with a race-effort workout or C-priority race.

You achieve the first objective by reducing the total work volume and including more recovery rides in the heart rate 1 zone. Reduce the duration of cruise intervals, maintaining muscular endurance, which has been a focus of training since Base 2. Something such as 4 or 5 × 3 minutes @ 4-5a (2 minutes @ 1) will stabilize this important element of racing fitness. By the weekend, you should be well rested and ready to go all out in a race or a race-effort workout. Table 6.12 suggests a training pattern that you can repeat in each Build R and R week.

Peak Period

Throughout the previous seven periods, training has become increasingly specific to the demands of racing. In the two-week Peak period, race specificity is the overriding focus. Reduce volume and space hard workouts further apart to allow more time for recovery. This last point is important as it means that you are fresher going into each tough session. Also in the Peak period, simulated races or actual races, especially the C-priority, end each week and serve as tune-ups before the real racing begins with A-priority events in the Race period.

There are two weekly workouts that you should do with racelike effort, as illustrated in table 6.13. For road racers and mountain bikers, one is continuing the SE intervals you did throughout the Build periods. One twist, however, is that the workout ends with a threshold ride, making it a stressful workout but one that closely simulates the effort necessary to race well. This workout may be something such as 5 × 2 minutes @ 5b (2 minutes @ 1) done on a steep hill, followed by 20 minutes in the heart rate 4-5a zones (20 minutes @ 4-5a). Mountain bikers should do this workout off road.

On the weekend, road racers include a race effort, group ride, or a race. In lieu of a race, mountain bikers ride off road

Table 6.13

TYPICAL PEAK PERIOD TRAINING WEEK

	Road racer	Mountain biker	Triathlete
Monday	Weights (PM phase)	Weights (PM phase)	Weights (PM phase) + swim
Tuesday	Sprints	Handling skills	Aerobic ride or run
Wednesday	AC intervals + threshold	AC intervals + threshold	Tempo brick + swim
Thursday	Recovery ride	Recovery road ride	Recovery ride or off
Friday	Day off	Day off	Day off or swim
Saturday	Aerobic ride	Aerobic ride	Aerobic run or ride
Sunday	Race effort or race	Race effort or race	Tempo brick or race

Table 6.14

TYPICAL RACE PERIOD TRAINING WEEK

	Road racer	Mountain biker	Triathlete
Monday	Day off	Day off	Swim
Tuesday	Aerobic ride	Aerobic road ride	Aerobic ride or run
Wednesday	Sprint + cruise intervals	Skills + cruise intervals	Tempo brick + swim
Thursday	Recovery ride	Recovery road ride	Recovery ride
Friday	Day off	Day off	Day off
Saturday	Aerobic ride or sprints	Aerobic ride or skills	Aerobic run or ride or brick
Sunday	Race	Race	Race

on a course that closely simulates the terrain expected in the upcoming A races. Include two or three time trials of about 20 minutes each on such a course, with 10 minutes of recovery between them, 3 × 20 minutes TT (10 minutes @ 1). This is best with another rider.

In addition to these workouts, road racers do a few match sprints early in the week. Something such as a few 15- to 20-second sprints with long recoveries will maintain power and sprint form. Mountain bikers can also include handling skills work.

If no race is available on the weekends, triathletes and duathletes may instead do race-tempo bricks for both their breakthrough workouts. One should be short, no longer than 90 minutes, and the other somewhat longer, at about one-half the longest race distance of the Race period. Do these at goal race pace. Triathletes may include a swim at the start of each brick, if the logistics of water and roads make it possible.

Race Period

Finally—it's time to race! This is when all the training time and hard work pay off. If you've been consistent in training for the preceding weeks, rested at the appropriate times, and cautiously apportioned workout intensity, you're in great shape and ready to perform at your best.

The only purpose of training in the Race period is to maintain fitness while resting between A-priority events. Omit weight training in A-race weeks to allow total recovery. Do one short muscular endurance workout at midweek to keep this key fitness element peaked. Carefully limit this to about 20 minutes total of race intensity. It could be something such as 5 × 3 minutes @ 4-5a (1 minute @ 1) for road racers and mountain bikers, or a short tempo brick for triathletes and duathletes. The only other hard workout is a race on the weekend. Many athletes find that a little race effort the day before a race helps prepare the body and mind for the next day's challenge. Others find that an easy workout, or even a day off, is best. Do what you know works for you. Table 6.14 suggests a Race week training pattern.

Making the Most of Race Day

At last race day arrives. This is the day for which you spent weeks preparing, physically and mentally. For an A-priority race, there was a long buildup followed by a period of tapering in which you came to a fitness peak. Along the way your life was molded around daily workouts. In the last few weeks you practiced the finer details of competition with simulations or tune-up races. You gave up many pleasures of life to prepare for this day. It would be a shame after all this preparation and sacrifice to make a mistake on race day and ruin the race, especially considering that you're going to peak only two or three times a season. There are several race-day details to consider; depending on your sport, some are more important than others.

Incredible fitness is not enough when your season goals are on the line. It's also necessary to have a race strategy for how you will expend energy in the event. Strategy is determined by several factors, such as course terrain, weather, other athletes including competitors and teammates, your strengths and weaknesses, and how training has gone in the previous days and weeks. Although these are important in every sport, some are more critical than others, depending on the type of event. For example, road racers must be outwardly focused on factors such as other competitors, and triathletes are mostly concentrating on their own strengths and weaknesses.

If you belong to a well-organized road-racing team, the group usually determines strategy in advance. Certain teammates may be protected as others are assigned to chase down breaks, lead the team's sprinters, or repeatedly test the other teams' resolve. Unfortunately, this kind of team cohesiveness and organization is rare in this country. For most masters road races, team strategy only includes not attacking a teammate, and even this basic rule is often violated. The wily road racer, however, will talk with teammates before the start to get organized. At the least, this means discussing the course, the competition, and what moves to expect. In American masters road racing, a well-conceived strategy can easily result in a single team determining the outcome of a race.

In mountain bike cross-country racing, strategy is largely an individual matter. The prerace decisions are based mostly on course layout and knowing how to pace yourself, especially early in the race when you are pumped up and fresh. Patience and conserving energy are important if you're to finish strongly. Mountain bike races have been described as "a time trial starting with a sprint." This is reasonably accurate given that starts are usually exceptionally fast, then the race settles down into a long, individual effort. To make matters worse, there is generally a long wait following the warm-up as the racers are staged. The mentally unprepared rider finds this frustrating and often wastes precious energy through increased nervous tension. The smart racer has prepared for this situation by physically practicing starts and mentally previewing how it will go. The resulting calmness means less fumbling for pedals and a better position early on.

Triathlon and duathlon racing is much like mountain biking, but with more emphasis on the time trialing and less on the starting sprint. In fact, the best strategy is to hold back in the early portion of the race. Finding your pace and holding it through each leg of the race is the most efficient use of energy. The longer the race, the more important such a strategy is. As in each sport, start discipline is part of the strategy. If you get caught in the excitement of the event and lose the necessary inward focus, chances are you'll be swept along at incredible speed for the first few minutes of the race, only to discover that you're deeply anaerobic with heavy breathing, lactate-drenched muscles, and a soaring heart rate. Such a mental breakdown has ruined many a race. If you're staying with the others in the initial minutes, chances are you started too fast. Once into the race, expend your energy in the most efficient manner. This means rationing the effort by watching your heart rate, listening to breathing, and monitoring perceived effort. Throughout the race, continually monitor your form and working muscles. Don't zone out—stay in tune with what's happening in your body. As with all good race strategies, you must practice this in training and tune-up races if you're to do it in the targeted events.

Race strategy includes determining food and fluid needs and scheduling feedings before and during the race. What will you eat for breakfast? Which sports drink will you use and how often? Should you take in solid food or gels during the race? When? Other considerations include the equipment you'll use, such as race wheels, gears, and special clothing. Then there are the details, such as what time you will arrive at the race venue, how you will prepare your bike and other equipment, and how you will warm up. You should have made these decisions days or even weeks before and practiced several times, especially during the Peak period.

Combining a well-designed and thoroughly practiced strategy with carefully considered goals and an effective annual plan that has brought you to a peak at just the right time is a great confidence builder and sure to produce the best performance possible. You're ready to race.

chapter

7

Rest and Recovery

The previous chapters suggested training programs for touring, century rides, and racing. All the workout regimens in those chapters are based on a normal recovery ability, but normal is a difficult concept to quantify in this context as we're each unique. This chapter will teach you how to rest, give you methods for recovery, and show you how to determine your individual needs.

The most important pieces of the training puzzle for the serious, past-50 rider are rest and recovery. Although all riders past the age of 50 know they don't recover as fast as when they were younger, there are still great individual differences. For one past-50 rider, a long ride on hilly terrain may require only two days of easy riding afterward, but for another it's three days, including one day entirely off the bike. To further complicate the matter, how fast you return to normal training differs from week to week within the same rider, depending on such variables as fitness level, recent diet, preceding workouts, and psychological stress.

Although restoration is a moving target, it's imperative to get it right. Cutting rest and recovery short just a few times is likely to result in overtraining, a weakened immune system, injury, loss of desire to ride, or chronic fatigue. Rest more than is necessary and you're wasting time, and possibly losing hard-earned fitness. Learning how to recover and how long to rest a past-50 body is the most important skill you can develop.

Recovery—Science to the Rescue

So how long should you recover, and what can you do to speed the process? Scientists have attempted to answer those questions, albeit with their fingers crossed. Let's look at what they've come up with in the two areas most closely related to recovery from hard rides—fatigue and muscle damage.

Fatigue—Friend and Foe

Fatigue is both friend and foe for the serious cyclist. On the one hand, it slows and even terminates rides. In extreme cases of fatigue, like after a fast century ride or hard-fought race, you may need several days to eliminate it. A purpose of training is to delay the onset of fatigue while improving the ability to cope with it. On the other hand, fatigue prevents a physiological catastrophe. Without such a regulating mechanism, the highly motivated rider would push to the point of destroying the body's cells, possibly resulting in permanent disability or even death. Whenever an organism faces internal threats to its health and stability, nature provides multiple restraint mechanisms. There are three such control devices affecting endurance cyclists that scientists have discovered and for which they've found coping strategies.

Beating the Burn

If you've been riding for 20 or more years, or you were an endurance athlete in another sport before it was fashionable, you probably have some misconceptions about lactic acid. Science once believed that it was responsible for a whole host of problems, the most notable of which was a delayed onset of muscle soreness following a hard ride. We now know that's not true. It is true, however, that the production of lactic acid causes fatigue. It would be more accurate to say that the b[inability to buffer or quickly remove lactate from the bloodstream causes fatigue. You may remember from chapter 3 that lactate is what lactic acid is called once it seeps through the muscle's cell walls into the blood. Once the muscles and blood are swimming in deep lactate, accompanied by localized muscle burning and labored breathing, reduced pedaling intensity is inevitable.

Once you reduce the pedaling intensity, lactate is quickly dispelled from the blood. With a decent cooldown, it's gone within an hour after getting off the bike. Lactate is not an issue for day-to-day recovery. It's strictly a short-term cause of fatigue. The next two fatigue agents are more insidious than the once-despised lactic acid.

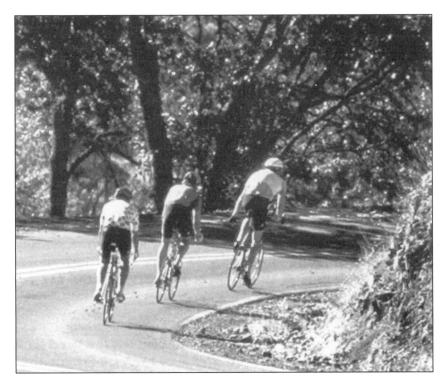

A long ride on hilly terrain may afterward require two days or more of easy riding.

Bonking Big Time

Endurance cycling events rely on both fat and glycogen for fuel. Glycogen is the form of carbohydrate stored in the muscles. At low-intensity riding, as in a tour, the ratio of fat to glycogen burned is 50-50, approximately equal amounts from both sources. As intensity increases, the volume of glycogen used for fuel increases relative to fat, so that during intense events, such as a criterium, glycogen is providing much of the energy. Although your body has enough stored fat to ride steadily for days, there is little glycogen, and because the body requires both be present, when glycogen runs out, the ride stops. Cyclists call this the bonk.

Once a bonk has occurred, recovery becomes a problem as it takes hours to replenish glycogen stores for the next ride. In fact, it's not necessary to bonk to face this recovery problem. A long or intense ride, especially early in the season when you haven't fully adapted to endurance riding, can bring glycogen levels to dangerously low levels. Eating carbohydrate under such conditions is imperative for recovery. If you do it right, recovery from glycogen depletion takes about 24 hours. This recovery rate is more dependent on fitness level than on age. In other words, a well-conditioned past-50 rider will spring back faster than a 30-year-old who is in poor shape.

Regardless of condition and age, the timing of carbohydrate ingestion is critical to this aspect of recovery. In the first few minutes after getting off the bike, there is the potential for a 300-percent increase in glycogen resynthesis, as compared with waiting two hours. This window of opportunity is the time to recover. Miss it following a particularly long or intense ride and you may require more than 24 hours to get back in the saddle. The details of this type of recovery process are explained shortly.

New and Improved Fatigue

Have you ever come in from a long ride and felt the need for a nap? If so, you've experienced a type of exercise fatigue that scientists have only recently discovered. What the folks in white lab coats found was that as muscles engaged in long endurance events use up a certain type of protein called branched-chain amino acids, the concentration of another amino acid, tryptophan, more than doubles. Once in the brain, tryptophan is converted to serotonin, a chemical that causes drowsiness. Now if you're trying to go to sleep at night, serotonin is a great thing to have lots of, but when riding it's a fatigue-producing nuisance. This persistent fatigue is common in riders in the advanced stages of overtraining. There is no known relationship of this type of fatigue to age. The key to breaking this cycle of increasing fatigue is as simple as maintaining adequate levels of branched-chain amino acids (BCAA) in your system, especially immediately following a long or intense ride. BCAA are found in foods high in quality protein.

That Darned Muscle Damage

Although lactate accumulation, energy depletion, and central nervous system fatigue are relatively short-term recovery issues, being fully resolved within 48 hours for most, damage to muscle is a different story. Following an intense ride, especially one that pushed you to the limits, some muscle membranes are mutilated. The longer the ride and the higher the intensity, the greater the damage. If you could peek into the muscles with a microscope following such a ride, you would see what looks like a battlefield with torn and leaking cells. The muscles most affected are of the fast twitch type, the ones that produce power. This damage causes soreness that begins within 8 to 12 hours and peaks by 24 to 48 hours. In the most severe cases the discomfort, decreased range of motion, and diminished strength aren't resolved for 72 hours and may last up to a week, although this is rare in cyclists.

Cannibalism

Such an intense ride has the potential to damage muscles another way. A hard ride can cause the loss of 30 grams of protein, about the amount in two cans of tuna. As the body turns to protein to provide a little fuel to augment fat and glycogen, muscle tissue is broken down. Scientists call this catabolism, but it could be called cannibalism. Without a strategy to replace this protein, especially in the face of closely spaced, repeated, intense efforts, wasting and loss of fitness is imminent. Limiting and quickly repairing such damage is critical for the serious cyclist.

Protein's Role

When it comes to repairing damaged muscle, protein is the key. Without adequate dietary levels of certain key protein building blocks that the body can't produce, recovery is delayed. These building blocks are the BCAA discussed earlier and must be present in the food you eat near the time of the workout to promptly repair the damage of a hard ride. BCAA are found in quality protein sources such as meat, poultry, fish, eggs, and dairy products, and, although not quite as absorbable by the body, in most vegetables and grains.

Science knows quite a bit about the protein recovery rate of young athletes. For example, one study looked at young male weightlifters and found that, with adequate amounts of quality protein, muscle repair happened rapidly. Four hours after a hard workout, protein synthesis was up about 50 percent higher than normal. By 24 hours it was elevated 109 percent, and returned to normal by 36 hours, indicating that the repair work was complete. Far less is known about what happens to the protein synthesis of past-50 riders, but from anecdotal evidence, it appears that recovery takes somewhat longer than this study found. That's all the more reason to focus on adequate protein before and after intense efforts.

Recovery Basics

As you can tell from the foregoing, the timing of carbohydrate and protein ingestion is critical to recovery following a stressful ride. Recovery begins well before getting on your bike, as early as two hours before, and continues for several hours after you get off. The following time schedule for recovery may seem overly detailed and structured, but if you are to achieve lofty goals, such a regimen will greatly improve your chances of success. The faster you recover, the sooner you can do another quality ride, and the quicker you get in shape.

This routine isn't necessary with all rides, just the intense and long ones that leave you wiped out. Here's a schedule of what to do before, during, and after a tough ride to speed recovery. As with anything new, try this fueling strategy in workouts before trying it in an important event.

Two hours before. The morning of a race, century, tour, or long or hard training ride, eat a breakfast no less than two hours before starting. This will top off the glycogen storage sites in your muscles and liver and provide a ready source of fuel floating around in the blood when it's time to ride. This meal should be high in carbohydrate, especially low-glycemic index carbohydrate. These are foods that release their energy slowly over several hours. Examples are apples, applesauce, grapefruit, peaches, pears, plums, milk, rye bread, sweet potatoes, tomato soup, and yogurt. (See chapter 9 for more details on glycemic index.) A little high-quality protein in this meal will provide the BCAA you need to limit muscle breakdown. This could be an egg or dairy product. The most important aspect of the preride meal is to eat what works for you. Don't eat anything that may cause you gastric distress later.

Once you've completed a meal two hours or more before starting the ride, don't take in anything other than water until just before the start. Some riders experience a low blood sugar reaction to carbohydrate consumed in the last 90 minutes.

Ten minutes before. Now is a good time to drink a high-glycemic index liquid such as a sports drink. This will ensure that you start the ride with fluid and fuel in your system. The sports drink you will use on the ride is good for this. A few swallows, up to about 12 ounces, will do the trick.

During the ride. For a ride lasting one hour or less, even an intense race like a criterium, water is sufficient, assuming you had an adequate meal two hours or more before. Beyond an hour, ingesting food, especially carbohydrate, plays an increasingly important role in recovery. The best way to get this carbohydrate is from standard commercial sports drinks, by slurping three to five ounces every 10 to 15 minutes during the ride. That's a little more than a 16-ounce bottle per hour. This aids recovery by sparing stored glycogen and muscle protein and reduces the need to wolf down copious quantities of food following the ride.

For intense rides lasting longer than three hours, swallowing gels or eating solid fuel in the form of energy bars or fruit provides a more condensed form of energy in addition to a sports drink. You may also find that mixing medium-chain triglycerides (MCT) into your sports drink provides an added boost to endurance and recovery. MCT is a form of fat that the body recognizes as similar to carbohydrate. It provides more energy per ounce than does carbohydrate, and you can purchase it in liquid form in many health food stores. Follow the directions on the label for mixing the liquid with a sports drink. MCT is a naturally occurring substance found in such foods as coconut oil and has no negative health effects.

Beyond six hours of riding demands that you include solid foods, such as sandwiches, cookies, energy bars, bagels, and fruit. High-glycemic index foods are still best. The lower intensity of such a ride makes digestion easier for solid foods. There's also good reason to believe that including BCAA for such long rides is beneficial. Commercial recovery drinks, such as Metabolol II, Pro Optibol, GatorPro, InterPhase, or Physique will provide these amino acids. Protein may also come from meat sources in the form of sandwiches, as eaten by riders in the Tour de France. A little fat in these feedings won't be a problem and may provide a feeling of satisfaction, allowing you to think less about your appetite and more about the ride.

Thirty minutes after. Within the first 30 minutes after getting off the bike, recovery swings into high gear. Due to the still-high blood flow to the legs and increased sensitivity of muscles to insulin, a storage hormone, your body is more ready to replace spent energy now than at any other time of the day. This is not the time for concern about losing weight. Failing to adequately refuel now means a longer recovery and less energy for riding in the ensuing 48 hours, as well as the possibility of a depressed immune system and a resulting cold.

Instead of dismounting and heading for the shower, head straight for the refrigerator. Studies have demonstrated that consuming carbohydrate, especially the high-glycemic index type, along with protein immediately following long and intense exercise is the best strategy. Mixing a little protein with the carbohydrate apparently causes the muscles to stock greater amounts of energy and restores essential proteins to muscles, allowing them to rebuild more quickly. You could accomplish this with either solid or liquid foods, but liquids are generally more appealing following a hard workout. Liquids also restore fluid levels. You'll need about .5 grams of carbohydrate and .2 grams of protein per pound of body weight at this time. Table 7.1 lists how many grams of each to have, based on various body weights.

One way to get this amount of carbohydrate and protein is

with a commercial recovery drink such as the ones listed in table 7.2. Owen Anderson, PhD, the publisher of Running Research News, suggests a recovery home brew, based on a study at the University of Florida by the scientist who created Gatorade. Anderson's drink provides the same benefits as the more expensive commercial products. To make your own home brew recovery drink, mix five tablespoons of sugar with 16 ounces of skim milk. Skim milk is used because fat delays digestion.

Table 7.1

CARBOHYDRATE AND PROTEIN NEEDS DURING RECOVERY BY BODY WEIGHT IN POUNDS

	BODY WEIGHT (LB)								
	120	**130**	**140**	**150**	**160**	**170**	**180**	**190**	**200**
Carbohydrate (g)	60	65	70	75	80	85	90	95	100
Protein (g)	24	26	28	30	32	34	36	38	40

Table 7.2

COMPARISON OF THE CARBOHYDRATE AND PROTEIN GRAMS OF POPULAR RECOVERY DRINKS

Drink	Carbohydrate	Protein
Endura Optimizer	59	11
GatorPro	65	19
InterPhase	81	36
Metabolol II	54	30
Met-Rx	18	32
Nitrofuel	75	11
Physique	86	32
ProOptibol	66	27
Home brew	60	13

All but home brew are based on 12 oz of solution when mixed with water. You can increase carbohydrate and protein concentrations by using milk or fruit juice instead of water or by blending in fruit. Twelve oz of skim milk, for example, adds 14 g of protein and 18 g of carbohydrate. A banana would add about 25 g of carbohydrate.

Two hours after. Within two hours after the ride, eat a meal that is mostly carbohydrate, but also includes quality protein, such as meat, fish, poultry, eggs, dairy products, or a combination of grains and beans. This meal keeps blood glucose and insulin levels high, encouraging the continued storage of glycogen while insulin sensitivity is still elevated. With another meal later in the day, you're well on the way to restocking energy and repairing muscle damage. The author of one study on nutrient recovery estimated that 40 to 50 percent of depleted glycogen stores can be resynthesized in the first six hours after a ride with proper eating (Ivy 1988). Within 24 hours you'll be close to preride levels, although not quite there, even if you did everything right. That's one reason for the hard day-easy day training system and spacing tough workouts by 48 hours or more.

Water is critical to recovery in the hours following a ride. Studies have shown that extreme perspiration can produce fluid losses of a half gallon per hour. Significant losses of body fluids greatly delay the recovery process. In the hours immediately following a hard ride, replace the water you lost by drinking liberally. To determine how much you need, weigh without clothes before and after a ride. The difference is mostly water loss. For every pound lost you need to drink about a pint of water.

Rest Is an Art Form

So far we've learned recovery tactics for returning the body to a normal state of readiness for the next ride. It's a process that follows all long or highly intense workouts throughout the year. Rest is a bit different. It's a planned strategy that's periodically applied to allow the body to absorb the training stresses and give you a mental break from the routine. Plan rest into your training within every week by setting aside one day for it. Include a week of rest in every three- or four-week training block during the Base and Build periods. Also, consider resting twice each year by taking a minivacation from training and doing something other than riding the bike. One of these Transition periods could come early in the summer and be one or two weeks long. For racers, this might come just

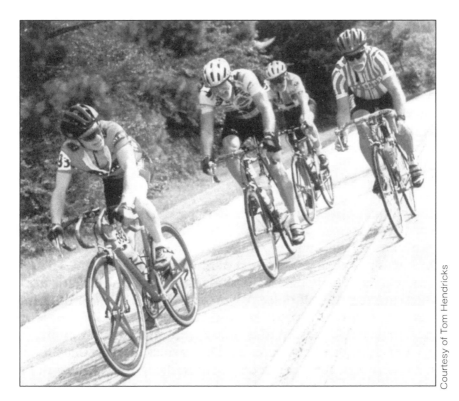

1997 Master National Road Race, Tallahassee, Florida

after the first peak. For century and tour riders, schedule it after a particularly difficult training period or following an event. Again, at the end of the riding season, plan a Transition period of three to six weeks.

Although rest may sound simple enough, there's actually quite a bit to it. Rest is both a science and an art, but mostly an art in that each rider has to determine the best form to apply. There are three forms of rest—active, passive, and therapeutic—from which to choose.

Active Rest

Sound like a contradiction? Not really, as some riders rest best with light activity. These are usually highly fit cyclists with many years on a saddle. For them, a short and easy spin at a low intensity (heart rate 1 zone or even less) provides many benefits, including a wave of fresh energy resources flowing to deep tissues, a reduction of soreness, lowered blood pressure, fresh air in the lungs, and a renewed outlook on life.

Active rest doesn't need to be on the bike. One of the best ways to rejuvenate with light activity is walking, especially in a wooded area or along the beach where the air is clean. Another that works wonders for some riders is exercising lightly in water. Floating in a swimming pool while gently moving the arms and legs is an effective form of active rest.

Passive Rest

Everyone, especially novice riders, but also experienced cyclists, needs time completely off the bike. No matter how fit and experienced you may be, there are times when you know the best thing is sitting on your duff and just enjoying life. There's a special joy that comes from total relaxation. The Italians have a saying for this: *Il dolce far niente,* the sweetness of doing nothing. Scientists know that total relaxation reduces the level of stress hormones in the blood and that this promotes a greater storage of glycogen in the muscles and reduces muscular tension. A day off after a particularly hard ride is not a waste of time, as some believe. It's another aspect of training.

Passive rest has been compared with the pauses that are an intricate part of a beautiful piece of music played by a well-conducted symphony. These absences of sound are what define the music. Without them, it would be just noise. In the same way, taking a periodic break from the bike makes for a sweeter symphony of fitness.

Therapeutic Rest

In addition to combining active and passive rest strategies, there are other approaches you can take to get the old body ready to ride again soon.

Sleep

There is nothing like sleep to rejuvenate the body. During a lengthy nap or night-long slumber, the pituitary gland at the base of the brain releases growth hormone. Growth hormone stimulates muscle growth and repair, bone building, and fat burning. It's a key hormone not only for recovery, but also for physiological improvement. Inadequate sleep means a diminished release of growth hormone and, ultimately, reduced performance on the bike. Growth hormone production diminishes with age, so paying close attention to rest becomes even more critical to success on the bike. Most past-50 riders need at least seven hours of sleep. When you have the time, a nap following a tough day on the bike will also boost your riding.

Massage

Most riders find that massage by an experienced massage therapist is a highly effective way to restore muscles, second only to sleep for its therapeutic benefits. Many riders believe, and some studies report, that massage improves psychological status, improves blood flow to muscles, relaxes muscle spasms, and relieves muscle pain. Within 24 to 36 hours following a hard ride, a massage therapist can work deeply in the tissues to provide these benefits.

Stretching

Gentle stretching in the hours following a ride helps nurse aching muscles back to normal by reducing the likelihood of an injury and speeding nutritional recovery. Stretching improves the rate at which muscles synthesize protein, a valuable aspect of recovery discussed earlier in this chapter. Chapter 8 covers stretching in greater detail.

Too Little, Too Late

Sometimes we're our own worst enemy. Riding and fitness are so much fun and become such high priorities that we cut back on rest to get a little more out of the old body. Or, we begin to feel invincible and don't pay enough attention to recovery. Then it happens: Overtraining, burnout, or illness strikes and we're on the sidelines watching.

Overtraining or Overliving?

Overtraining is a physical condition primarily marked by a chronically reduced capacity for work, brought on by an imbalance between stress and rest. The stress can come in several forms and is not limited to training. Other stress producers that may cause overtraining are lifestyle related, such as working too much or eating an inadequate diet. Psychological stress, like financial worries or marital problems, is often overlooked as a cause of poor riding performance. In fact, training may be a minor player in the overtraining scenario and yet be the aspect of life in which the condition is most obvious. Because a combination of too much stress from any aspect of life can result in overtraining, a more appropriate name for the condition might be overliving.

Overtraining can happen to any rider at any age, but past-50 cyclists, as a group, seem less susceptible, as they are a little wiser when it comes to balance in life. That doesn't mean it can't or won't happen to you.

The most noticeable symptom of overtraining is poor riding performance. Work output (speed) is low compared with work

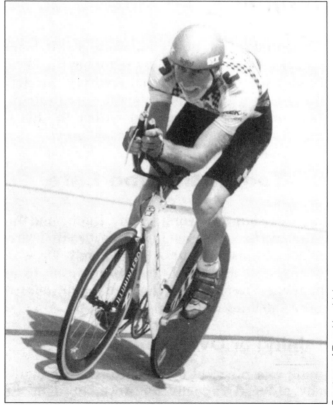

Courtesy of Tom Hendricks

Tom Hendricks at 3000 Track Pursuit, Masters National Track 1997.

input (effort). Other signs are often present telling you that something isn't right. Common secondary indicators include weight change, heart rate deflections, muscle or joint soreness, swollen lymph glands, diarrhea, slow-healing wounds, irritability, poor sleep patterns, and sluggishness.

The best prevention for this condition, as you might have guessed, is adequate and well-timed rest and recovery. The more stress producers in your life, the greater the need for R and R. Highly motivated riders are at the greatest risk. They deal with reduced performance by pushing themselves harder and thus compound the problem. This is the best reason for having a coach or trainer as an experienced and unbiased observer. A coach is usually a better judge of a rider's needs than is the rider.

If you suspect overtraining, train alone for two or three days at a low intensity, such as the heart rate 1 zone. It is often best to do this training in a mode other than bicycling. Swimming is the best option. Avoid working out with other riders as the competitive zeal may elevate the intensity. If the symptoms persist after three days of easy training, take two to five days of complete rest. That means no riding no matter how low the intensity is and reducing all physical stress. Get extra sleep, take naps, stay off your feet, and pursue other pleasures in life. If not improved after five additional days off the bike, see your doctor. He or she may call for a blood test to look for unusual cell counts or general chemistry abnormalities. Should you experience illness at any time, see your doctor right away.

Burnout

Competition has an emotional cost. Every time you ride in an event in which a comparison with others is a strong element, whether such ranking is inherent to the event or self-imposed, you leave some portion of your emotional makeup behind. Riders with years of experience are more hardened to competition, so have a lower emotional price to pay than those new to the sport. After some number of competitions, without a rest break separating them, a rider burns out.

Burnout is also common to the compulsive rider. Endurance sports such as cycling often attract people who are internally driven, or obsessed, by their activity. There is a thin line that separates compulsion from motivation, but the difference is evident in the rider who can't take a day off or feels overwhelmed by guilt when he or she does. Cyclists who keep records of how many days they've gone without missing a ride are probably compulsive. Obsessive-compulsive behavior often leads to burnout in such people, but they continue to ride despite declining enthusiasm and waning performance.

Burnout is marked by a mental slump that has no obvious physical symptoms. There is a decreased interest in competition, and just getting on the bike for an easy spin requires great fortitude. Riding becomes drudgery. Slight weather variations from the norm, such as heat or light rain, become overwhelming obstacles to getting on the bike. The burned-out rider has low motivation to succeed at anything, and enthusiasm for life is lacking. To make matters worse, the burned-out cyclist second guesses the decision not to ride on a given day, so lowered self-confidence grows. The downward spiral eventually causes a mental crash, forcing extended time off the bike. Some never recover and give up riding. Others return to the sport in a few weeks or months with renewed enthusiasm but a greatly diminished capacity for exercise.

As with overtraining, the best cure for burnout is prevention. Weekly, monthly, and annual rest breaks recharge the batteries and keep riding in perspective. Especially effective is the twice-annual Transition period described earlier. A week or two away from riding early in the summer and three to six weeks off in the late fall is potent medicine for burnout. When you suspect burnout, the only cure is rest. Stay away from the bike until you itch to get back on.

Illness and Riding

Upper respiratory infections such as head colds and sore throats are all too common with riders, especially in the days following an extremely trying event or workout. The six hours after such a ride are the most critical, as the immune system is depressed. This is when you're most likely to catch a cold. Studies have demonstrated that athletes who train at high workloads are twice as likely to be sick as those who train at relatively low workloads.

What should you do when illness first shows up? Should you continue to train as normal or completely rest? One way to answer that question is to do a neck check. If the symptoms are above the neck, like runny nose or nasal congestion, it probably won't do you any harm to ride, as long as the workout is low intensity and the duration is short. Symptoms below the neck, including chest congestion, achy muscles, and fever, are a sure sign that you need a day off. Trying to train through such an illness could easily set you up for far worse complications, such as an inflammation of the heart or lungs caused by a virus or bacteria.

At the first sign of a cold, pamper your body by increasing rest and decreasing stress of all types. Drinking fluids, taking vitamin C, and sucking on zinc lozenges all reduce the severity and duration of cold symptoms in athletes.

When the symptoms finally abate and it's time to start training again, you may notice a loss of strength and aerobic capacity that lasts a few days up to several weeks, depending on how severe the illness was. While getting back to normal, it's best to train with caution, reestablishing the basic elements of fitness, such as aerobic and muscular endurance, and strength. One way to do this is to return to the Base period of training for two days for every day you had symptoms.

Rest and Recovery in the Real World

It should be apparent by now that for the past-50 rider, rest and recovery are every bit as important for fitness as riding the bike, if not more so. The only problem with rest and recovery is knowing exactly when and how to fit them in. Unfortunately, no one can tell you that; you must discover it for yourself. The way to find your unique rest and recovery needs is by listening to your body. By the age of 50, most experienced riders are pretty good at that, but some aren't.

Recent research from Australia reveals that monitoring sleep quality, fatigue, stress, and muscle soreness can help predict when you need more rest. Other indicators of the need to cut back could be waking heart rate and body weight. Check each warning sign within the first 30 minutes after waking. Rate sleep, fatigue, stress, and muscle soreness on a scale of one to seven, with one being the best situation and seven the worst. Record these in your training log along with resting heart rate as beats higher or lower than your normal waking pulse, and body weight as pounds higher or lower than normal. Establish these norms during a period of light training when you are well rested.

Rating any of these as five or higher is a warning sign that you need more rest. Such a morning warning indicates the need for active, passive, or therapeutic rest. Three such morning warnings are a sure sign that you need a day off.

This ranking system isn't foolproof. There will be days when you talk yourself out of high ratings to ride as planned and others when you'll forget or won't have time. Listening intently to what your body is saying daily, however, has great potential to help the past-50 cyclist stay in tune with rest and recovery needs. When unsure about what course of action to take on any day, the best advice is to opt for more rest and recovery. When in doubt—leave it out.

chapter

8

Avoiding Injury

Passing the 50-year mark has both good and bad sides. The greatest advantage of aging is wisdom resulting from an accumulating body of knowledge seasoned by years of experience. Veteran cyclists are worldly wise when it comes to understanding their bodies. The worst of the downside from a half-century of living is the propensity for aches and pains. For past-50 cyclists, some nagging injuries are simply part of the deal—things are more likely to break down and need maintenance the older one gets. Other physical problems, perhaps most for the otherwise fit and healthy veteran, are a direct result of saddle time. Wisdom doesn't mean omnipotence; we still make mistakes in training.

We can divide cycling-related breakdowns by cause into extrinsic and intrinsic injuries. Extrinsic includes those injuries resulting from sudden events, such as crashes and muscles torn while sprinting. These are the kind veteran cyclists are pretty good at avoiding. The other category, intrinsic, are much more insidious and likely to plague the veteran. Three types of intrinsic injuries sneak up on the unsuspecting cyclist. The first type relates to the environment of cycling. An incorrect bike setup is the most common example here, but another is an inadequate diet. The second type has to do with hereditary factors, such as a leg-length discrepancy or chronically tight hamstrings. The third is training related. Incorrect training methods generally mean doing too much, too soon. Given small enough increases in workload over a long enough time, the body will adapt and grow strong and resilient. Try to rush it, and problems result. All cycling injuries common to the past-50 cyclist can be cured, and better yet, prevented. Let's look at prevention first.

Staying Healthy

Some past-50 cyclists have bodies of steel. They can get away with almost anything and never have an injury. Others seem to be made of glass. The slightest mistake in training means another injury. If you are in this latter group, you must do whatever it takes to stay healthy. Here are five suggestions for avoiding injury.

Overreaching

As discussed in chapter 3, the purpose of training is to slightly overload the body's systems to produce a training effect. Going beyond what you need for this adaptive process is called overreaching. We can compare it with wasting money. When buying a new car you wouldn't think of offering the salesperson $100 more than the asking price, yet when it comes to training, riders frequently do the physical equivalent of that. If two hours are all you need, some will ride three. If five intervals will achieve the benefit, many do six. More is seldom better, and is often worse.

The most important aspect of staying out of your doctor's office is moderation. If you regularly push to your physical limits and beyond, the risk of injury skyrockets. The idea is to always do a little less than you think is possible, saving something for another day. For example, when doing intervals you probably know when there is only one left in you. That's the time to stop. Always finish knowing you could have done a few more miles, one more interval, another hill or two, and a couple more reps in the weight room.

The same goes for planning annual hours, if you're following a racing program like the one described in chapter 6. Increases in the hours trained from one year to the next should be no greater than 10 percent, and 5 percent is better. Biting off more than you can chew when planning the race season means chronic fatigue and raises the specters of overtraining, burn-out, illness, and injury.

Warm-Up and Cooldown

When you were in school 30 to 40 years ago, you warmed up before a physical education class or sports practice with calisthenics. Regardless of the activity, you stood in rank and file and did such things as toe touches, jumping jacks, bend and reach, and windmills. Warming up this way wasn't all that bad, as at least it got the blood flowing, and for the supple body you had then, a lot of mistakes could be made. Now you know that jumping jacks, although not terrible, are not the best way to prepare for a bike ride. You also can no longer afford to make any mistakes, especially when the planned ride is intense, such as intervals, hills, or a race.

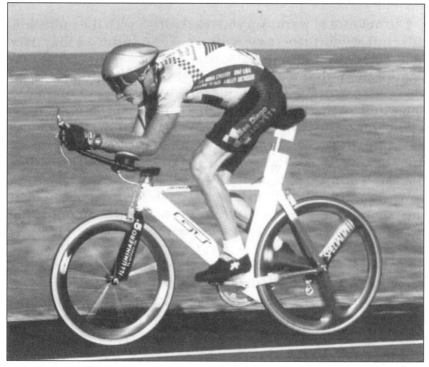

Moriarty, New Mexico. Tom Hendricks setting the national time trial record for the 60-64 age group in 1997.

Proper warm-up has many benefits that prevent major injuries, especially the extrinsic type, but also help avoid the intrinsic, overuse injuries that crop up regularly. These benefits include

- thinning body fluids to allow easier muscle contraction and less work for the heart,
- opening capillaries to bring more oxygen to the working muscles,
- sensitizing the nervous system for smoother movements,
- decreasing stress on the heart and muscles,
- raising muscle temperature so contractions are more rapid,
- conserving carbohydrate and releasing fat for fuel,
- reducing initial levels of lactic acid, and
- helping asthmatics avoid constriction of airways.

The amount of warm-up you need varies with the individual rider but seems to increase with age. Young athletes may need only 10 minutes of warm-up, whereas a past-50 cyclist may require twice that for the same benefits. Warm-up duration also varies with the type of ride for which you're preparing. A short and intense ride, such as intervals or a criterium, needs a long warm-up. Long, low-intensity rides require only a short warm-up, if any. The cooler the weather, the longer the warm-up. The inverse of this is also true. The warmer the weather, the less warm-up you need.

Warm-up duration is an individual matter. Not only do some riders need more or less than others, but the amount that riders can tolerate is largely determined by aerobic and muscular endurance levels. A rider with an excellent base of fitness who is well adapted to long endurance rides has the capacity to warm up longer than one whose fitness is less developed. As a rule, the combined time of the warm-up, the intense portion of the workout, and the cooldown should not exceed 50 percent of your most recent longest ride.

During the course of several minutes, the warm-up should build from low effort in the heart rate 1 zone to moderate effort in the heart rate 3 zone. This may take 10 to 20 minutes or more for some riders. Once you have achieved the 3 zone, continue the warm-up with several short accelerations, per-haps 10- to 30-seconds duration each. The intensity of these is the effort you anticipate in the ensuing workout or race, using the gearing combination you plan for the event. Recover for a minute or two after each acceleration by riding slowly in a low gear.

Ideally, the workout or race should start no more than a minute or two following the last acceleration, because you rapidly lose the warm-up benefits with inactivity. Although you can easily control such tight timing in a workout, it is seldom possible before a race starts.

If you race, design and regularly practice a warm-up proce-dure in workouts so that on race day it is automatic. With the many distractions before a race start, you want to have the routine nailed down.

Although cooldown following an intense ride is seldom critical for avoiding injury, it does assist with recovery. Studies have shown that 20 minutes of easy riding returns blood lactate levels to near resting levels, but that abruptly stopping an intense ride clears only half the lactate within 20 minutes.

Stretching

Most veteran riders talk about stretching with an almost mystical reverence, especially when they're injured. "I haven't been stretching enough," is a common explanation for a sore hamstring or achy back. Although stretching is helpful in injury prevention, lack of it is seldom the only cause of a breakdown. On the other hand, the loss of range of motion that accompanies aging can contribute to an injury, both of the extrinsic and intrinsic types. You can reverse this loss of flexibility, which begins as early as the fourth decade of life, with daily stretching, especially following a ride while the muscles are still pliable. If not periodically stretched, connec-tive tissues become more dense and less stretchable.

There is a great deal of individual variance in flexibility due to differences in the positioning of muscle attachments to tendons and bones. Riders who can, for example, touch the ground with their fingers while standing without bending their knees probably have less need for stretching than those who have a hard time touching their knees in this position.

Although the latter are in greater need of flexibility to prevent injury, they seldom do it because of the discomfort that accompanies stretching.

Another reason past-50 cyclists often give for a reluctance to begin a stretching routine is that they believe positive changes are unlikely at their age. Research has demonstrated, however, that you can improve range of motion at any age. One study found that stretching produced the same percent improvement in people aged 63 to 88 as in teenagers.

Stretching methods have changed in the last 30 years. In the 1960s, ballistic stretching with rapid, bobbing movements was popular. This technique is likely to produce a reduced range of motion, because stretch receptors in the tissues feed a signal back to the muscle to tighten in order to prevent a tear when rapidly stretched. In the 1970s a Californian by the name of Bob Anderson wrote a book called *Stretching* that ushered in a new way of improving flexibility. Anderson's technique, known as *static stretching*, is still the most common method used by athletes in many sports, including cycling. In static stretching you hold a position for several seconds as you allow the muscle to relax. The duration of a static stretch is generally less than a minute, with 10 to 30 seconds most common.

About the same time static stretching became popular among athletes, another technique was gaining support in the scientific literature. *Proprioceptive neuromuscular facilitation*, also thankfully called PNF stretching, is based on the principle that a muscle more completely relaxes after a powerful contraction. The contraction can involve tightening either the stretched muscle or its antagonist (the muscle on the opposite side of the limb is an antagonist). Either way, the PNF technique has proven 10 to 15 percent more effective in loosening muscles than static stretching.

To PNF stretch the hamstrings, for example, you first static stretch the muscle for 8 to 10 seconds, then relax it while contracting the quadriceps on the front of the leg for 8 to 10 seconds, and finally static stretch the hamstrings again. Or, you could static stretch the hamstrings for 8 to 10 seconds, then isometrically contract the hamstrings for 8 to 10 seconds, followed by a static stretch of the hamstrings again. In either case, repeat the routine three times for each muscle group you stretch.

Whichever method you prefer to use, static or PNF, the best time to stretch is following a ride. An exception is a tight lower back, which you should loosen up before starting a ride. Stretching after a workout hastens the recovery process by encouraging muscles to replenish glycogen stores quickly and speeding protein synthesis needed for muscle repairs following strenuous rides. The muscle groups most in need of stretching following a ride are the calf, hamstring, quadriceps, gluteus, lower back, upper back, and neck. Figure 8.1 illustrates how to stretch these muscle groups.

Strength

Aging is typically accompanied by a loss of muscle mass and bone density, although the more active you are, the smaller the losses. Shrinking muscles increase the likelihood of injury and

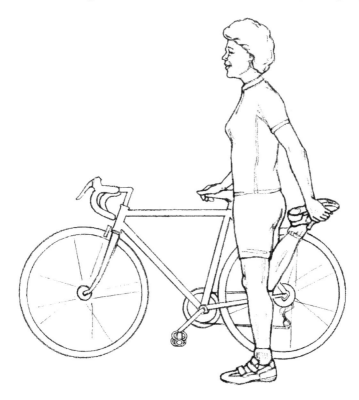

(continued)

Figure 8.1 Routine for postride stretching

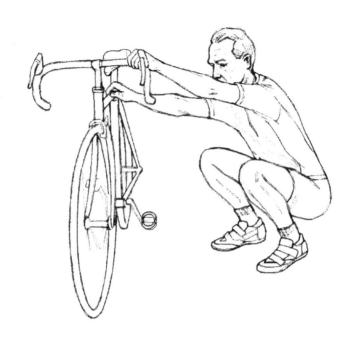

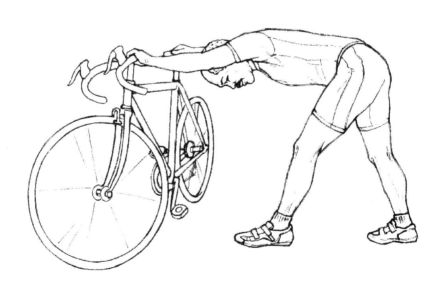

Figure 8.1 *(continued)*

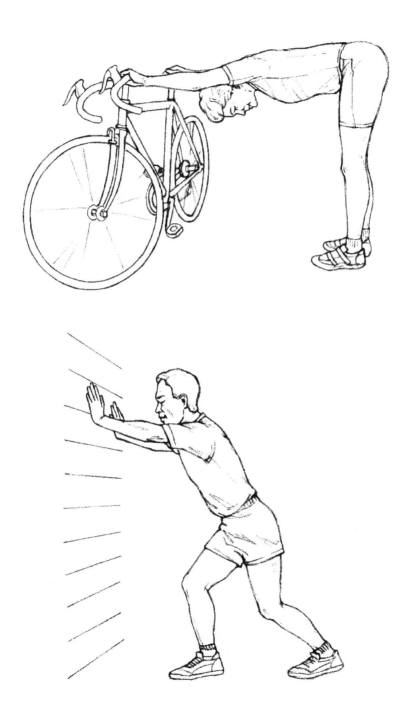

Figure 8.1 *(continued)*

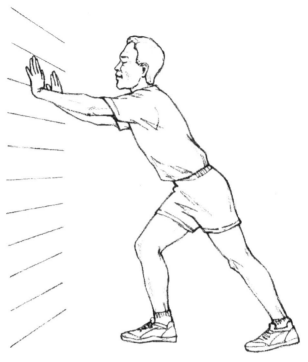

Figure 8.1 *(continued)*

mean reduced power and strength for sprinting and climbing. Reduced bone health is especially worrisome.

Cycling is a great sport for maintaining lower body muscles and bones, but does little for the upper body. That may lead to problems later in life, especially by raising the specter of osteoporosis. Weight training is one solution. A few years ago, a university study conducted with subjects aged 55 and older found that combining weight training with a vigorous walking program improved bone density in both the upper and lower body areas.

Besides improving muscle mass and bone density above the waist, weight training strengthens the muscles, tendons, and ligaments of the foot, ankle, knee, and hip joints so important to cycling. It can also correct imbalances and improve the range of motion of joints. All this means a lower risk of injury in the short term and later in life.

Rules to Lift By

There are as many different weight-training programs as there are coaches and trainers. It's doubtful that any, including the one suggested here, exactly meets your unique needs. Some experimentation may be necessary to discover that. Even if you never find, or even look for, the perfect program, it's important to simply start strength building. Lifting weights has great benefits for the aging cyclist, irrespective of routines, sets, repetitions, and loads. There are, however, certain considerations in weight training that will allow you to get more benefit for cycling performance from any program. The following rules to lift by guide you in becoming a stronger and more injury-resistant cyclist. You will not bulk up and look like a bodybuilder by lifting weights according to these rules.

- Rule 1. Train the big muscles. The big muscles are in the thighs, butt, calves, back, abdomen, and chest. It's best to work these major movers with free weights whenever possible, as they force you to maintain balance, which also strengthens the smaller, supportive muscles. For some exercises, such as the lat pull, free weights aren't practical, however. Also, if you have a joint, such as a knee, that is inherently weak from prior injuries, you may be better off using a machine for stability.

- Rule 2. Use multijoint exercises. A multijoint exercise is one that involves two or more joints within the same movement. For example, a seated knee extension works the quadriceps muscle on the front of the thigh, but uses only the knee joint. The squat also works the quadriceps, while including the knee, hip, and ankle. Because you use so many joints, you work more muscles at the same time. Besides the quadriceps, the squat exercise also strengthens the hamstrings, calf, gluteus, and lower back. This not only saves you time in the weight room, but also develops your muscles in a way similar to how you use them on the bike. You never extend your knee on the bike without also involving the muscles of the hip and ankle.

- Rule 3. Mimic the positions of cycling. In doing the squat, place the feet the same width apart as the pedals on your bike with your feet pointed straight ahead. Why? Because you want the strength you develop to transfer to useable strength when you ride. Your pedals aren't shoulder-width apart, and your feet don't point out or in when pedaling. In the same way, grip bars and machines as though holding your handlebars whenever possible. The more bikelike your strength training is, the more cycling-related benefits you'll reap.

- Rule 4. Keep the number of exercises low. Focus on several sets in a few, key exercises, rather than a shotgun approach with many exercises and limited sets of each. By using multijoint movements, you can greatly reduce the number of exercises you do in the weight room. That means less time lifting, and more time riding or with your family. Figures 8.2 through 8.7 illustrate nine exercises that follow these rules.

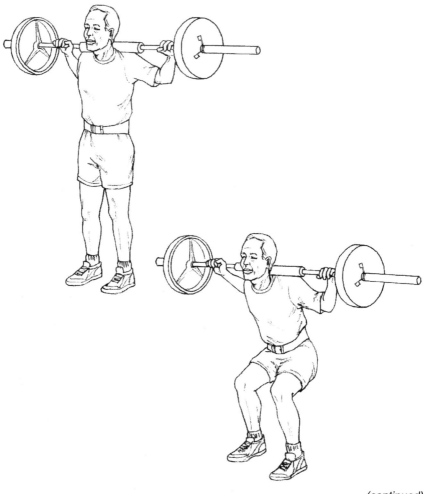

Figure 8.2 Hip extension

(continued)

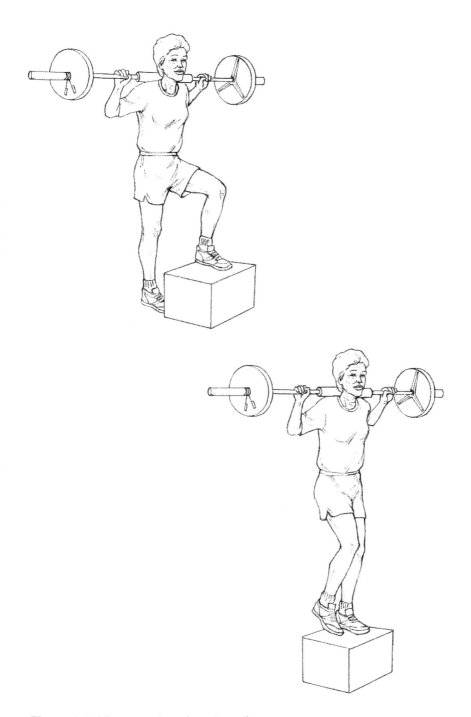

Figure 8.2 Hip extension *(continued)*

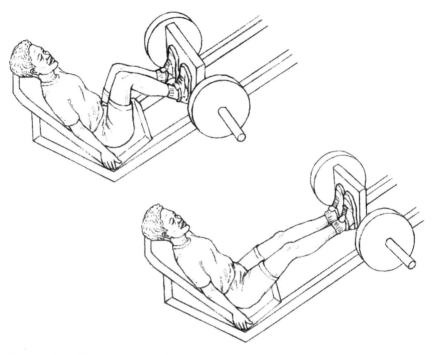

Figure 8.2 Hip extension *(continued)*

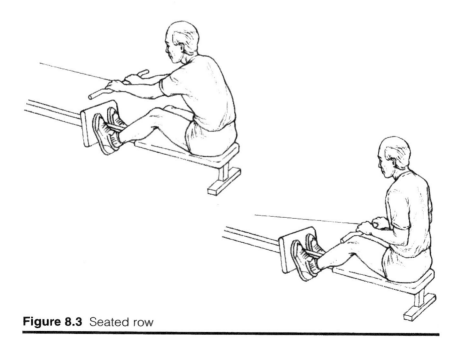

Figure 8.3 Seated row

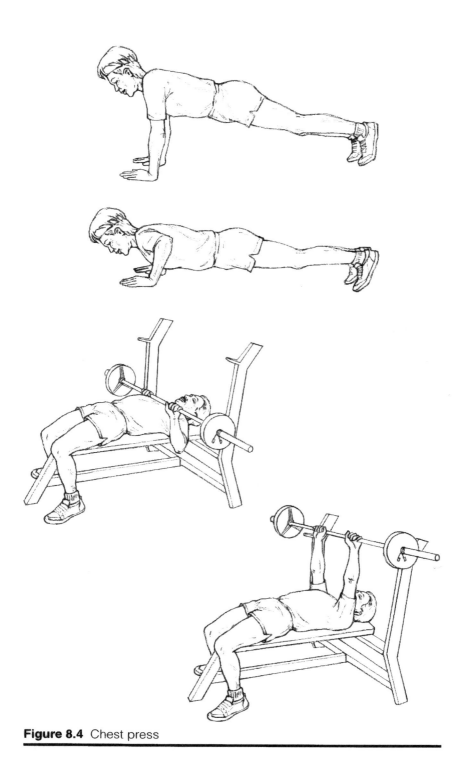

Figure 8.4 Chest press

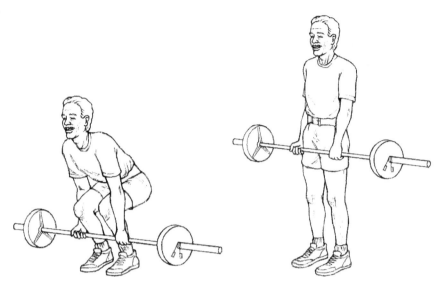

Figure 8.5 Dead lift

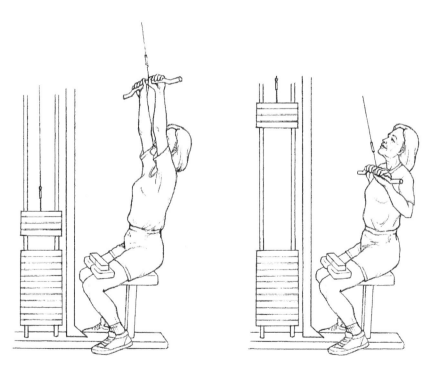

Figure 8.6 Lat pull

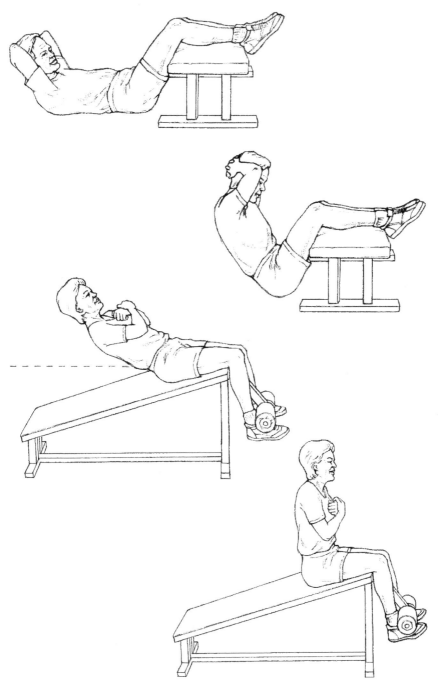

Figure 8.7 Abdominal

Strength Phases

There are six phases of strength training that coincide with the buildup to your event, whether it's a race, century, or tour. The six phases are explained here and summarized in table 8.1.

Anatomical Adaptation (AA) phase. The purpose of this phase is to strengthen muscles and tendons throughout the body in preparation for the greater loads of the next phase known as Maximum Strength. Start loads cautiously low in the first week of this phase and increase weekly, perhaps with every session. Other than toughening connective tissues, it's also important to refine the movements of each exercise by lifting slowly, emphasizing perfect form.

Maximum Strength (MS) phase. This is the key phase in strength training. The stronger you become now, the greater will be your gains in the later phases. Lifting heavy weights challenges both the muscular and the nervous systems by teaching them to recruit most, if not all, available muscles to lift the weight. Both the endurance-important, slow twitch muscles and the fast twitch, power muscles are strengthened. Start the first session of this phase with a conservative load, but challenge yourself regularly to increase the weight. Movements are slow to moderate, emphasizing perfect form. Be cautious in this phase. If your knees or other joints don't feel right in some exercise, reduce the load, change the exercise, or omit that movement.

Power Endurance (PE) phase. In this phase you will convert the strength and ability to recruit large numbers of muscle fibers from the MS phase to sport-specific power by combining force with speed. Reduce loads to moderate levels for fast movement. Do quick, explosive action only as you lift the weight, but set it down slowly. Don't move so rapidly that you lose control of the weight. You need long rests between sets in this phase as the nervous system is slow to recover. You may think your muscles are ready to go again, but the nerves aren't.

Muscular Endurance (ME) phase. The first change you will notice in the phase, with its high repetitions and light loads, is a burning sensation in the muscles you work. That's a result of accumulating lactate. The ME phase will help your muscles learn to deal with such fatigue by increasing capillary density and the number and size of energy production sites called

STRENGTH PHASES

	AA	MS	PE	ME	SM	PM
Weeks per phase						
Novice	8-10	3-4	3-4	6-8	2-3	2-3
Experienced	4-6	4-6	4-6	6-8	2-3	2-3
Days per week						
Novice	2-3	2	2	1-2	1-2	1-2
Experienced	2-3	2	2	1-2	1-2	1-2
Exercises* (in order of completion)						
Novice	1-2-3-4-6-7	1-6-2-7	1-6-2-7	1-6-2-7	1-6-2-7	1-6-2-7
Experienced	1-2-3-4-5-6-7	1-6-2-7	1-6-2-7	1-6-2-7	1-6-2-7	1-6-2-7
Load (% of 1RM)						
Novice	40-60	80-90	30-50	30-50	60, 60, 80	30-50
Experienced	40-60	85-95	40-60	30-50	60, 60, 80	40-60
Sets						
Novice	3	3-4	3-4	2-3	2-3	1-2
Experienced	3-5	4-8	3-5	3-4	2-3	2-3
Repetitions per set						
Novice	20-30	4-8	8-15	40-60	6-12	8-15
Experienced	20-30	3-6	8-15	40-60	6-12	8-15
Speed of movement						
Novice	Slow	Slow to moderate	Fast	Mod	Slow to moderate	Fast
Experienced	Slow	Slow to moderate	Fast	Mod	Slow to moderate	Fast
Recovery between sets (min)						
Novice	1-1.5	2-4	3-5	1-2	1-2	3-5
Experienced	1-1.5	2-4	3-5	1-2	1-2	3-5

*Exercise 1-hip extension (squat, step-up, or leg press), 2-seated row, 3-hip extension (different from 1), 4-chest press (bench press or push-up), 5-dead lift, 6-seated lat pull to chest, 7-abdominal (for abdominal, always use AA load, reps, sets, recovery, and speed regardless of phase) mitochondria. Keep recoveries between sets short to further encourage these changes.

Strength Maintenance (SM) phase. After a long ME phase, it's time to rebuild your strength, only now with somewhat lighter weights and higher repetitions, because your event is approaching and you have increased riding intensity. Do two or three sets for each exercise once or twice a week. The first set or two are for warm-up only. For the last set increase the load to about 80 percent of maximum for 8 to 12 repetitions. When you can do 12 repetitions, increase the weight in your next session.

Power Maintenance (PM) phase. This repeats the PE phase you did earlier in the season, only this time you may reduce days per week and sets to maintenance levels. Again, be cautious in this phase with speed of movement. Always keep the weight under control.

Periodization of Strength

Just as in training on the bike, strength training should follow the, concept of periodization. By periodically changing the emphasis in the weight room, your body will reap different benefits, and you'll avoid overuse injuries. Table 8.2 suggests how to blend strength and bike training into a periodization plan.

Table 8.2

PERIODIZATION OF STRENGTH PHASES FOR RACE, CENTURY, AND TOUR TRAINING

	RACE	CENTURY	TOUR
Phase	**(Period)**	**(Period)**	**(Weeks prior)**
AA	Prep	Period 1	23-26
MS	Base 1	Period 2	19-22
PE	Base 2	Period 3	15-18
ME	Base 3, Build 1	Period 4-5	7-14
SM	Build 2-3	Period 6	4-6
PM	Peak	Period 6	2-4

Determining Loads

Perhaps the most difficult aspect of weight training is figuring out how much weight to use for each exercise within each phase. One way of doing this is to test your strength at the start of each new phase to see how much weight you can lift one time. This is called a one-repetition maximum, often abbreviated as 1RM, and is a simple way of determining loads. You may have noticed, in fact, that the loads listed in table 8.1 are based on percentages of 1RM. The problem with this method is that such a test can leave you so sore for the next two days that you're unable to ride or even do simple tasks around the house. The risk of injury is also high. For these reasons, I don't recommend determining loads in this manner.

A less risky method estimates 1RM based on doing a higher number of repetitions to near failure. Start by doing a warm-up set or two of the exercise you will measure. Then select a weight you can lift at least 4 times, but no more than 10. You may need to experiment for a couple sets. If you do, rest for five minutes between attempts. To find your predicted 1RM, divide the weight lifted by the factor in table 8.3 that corresponds with the number of repetitions lifted. For example, if you could manage six repetitions with a load of 150 pounds, you can find your estimated 1RM by dividing 150 by .85. Your 1RM is 175, in this case.

Another and simpler way to estimate the load to use in any phase is to guess, based on experience, then adjust the weight as you progress. This is probably the most commonly used

Table 8.3

PREDICTING 1RM

Number of reps	Factor
4	.90
5	.875
6	.85
7	.825
8	.80
9	.775
10	.75

method of load determination. If you find load this way, be especially conservative at the start of the MS and PE phases. Better to start too light than too heavy.

Aches and Pains of Excellence

No matter how well you warm up, stretch, and strengthen muscles, you're likely to experience a bike-related injury. Striving for excellence in cycling means that you will frequently approach your physical limits on the bike, and from time to time there will be little aches and pains that come and go. Some stay longer than others and affect not only your riding, but also your daily activities at times. These are injuries.

The most common site of pain for cyclists is the knee. There are several possible injuries to the knee, including chondromalacia patella, patella tendinitis, iliotibial band inflammation, and tendinitis of the hamstring attachments behind the knee. Other common injuries caused by riding are Achilles tendinitis; tingling or numb hands; and pain in the neck, back, and elbows. It's a rare cyclist who has never experienced one of these.

Injury Assessment

When soreness develops you need to pay close attention to it. Determine exactly where the discomfort is. Can you put a finger on the spot or is it more general? Write in your training log when any discomfort begins, no matter how trivial it may seem at the time. This could be valuable information later as you're trying to remember exactly when a bad injury started and what may have caused it.

The intrinsic types of injuries most common in cycling come on slowly over several days or weeks. These are typically classified as overuse injuries and progress through four stages, or grades of severity.

Grade I Injuries

The lowest level of injury is a grade I. At this initial stage you may experience only discomfort, not pain, after getting off the bike. This discomfort typically continues for several hours

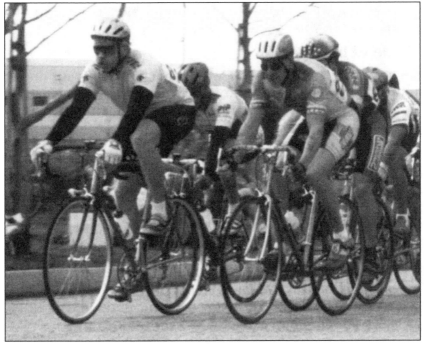

Courtesy of Peter Weiner

After any race, fill up on rest and recovery.

before slowly fading away. At this level of injury you should seek and eliminate the cause while training cautiously. How to determine causes is explained shortly.

Grade II Injuries

The injury is now a little worse. You experience some discomfort, which you still would not classify as pain, during a ride. The discomfort may disappear when you're well warmed up, only to reappear after the ride. It's not bad enough to affect your riding. Again, deal with this by seeking and eliminating the cause. If the discomfort persists for two weeks, reduce your training volume and intensity and see a doctor.

Grade III Injuries

You've not been listening to your body. Pain now occurs during a ride and causes you to favor the affected area by gear selection, shifting on the saddle, or altering pedaling technique. Greatly reduce your training and cross train, but don't do anything that aggravates the injury site. Determine the cause and see your doctor.

Grade IV Injuries

You're unable to ride. You've waited too long. See your doctor immediately. Stay off the bike, but investigate the cause while cross-training in a way that doesn't cause further damage.

Treat the Cause

No matter how slight or severe the injury may be, the first thing you must always do is determine what caused it. Until you know this, treatment will only deal with the symptoms, but the injury will keep returning. The following questions will help you find the cause and eliminate it.

- Did the injury come on gradually or suddenly? If it was gradual, it is probably related to small changes that occurred either in your bike, training, or body. The cause for a sudden injury is usually easy to pinpoint.
- Has this ever happened before? Assuming you noted this in your training journal, what did you do about it then? Is the injury more or less severe than it was the last time?
- Have you recently changed training methods? Are you riding more miles or putting in longer rides than your body was ready for? Has the intensity of your training increased too rapidly by riding hills or doing hard rides?
- Have you recently changed the phase of your strength program, especially to the Maximum Strength or Power Endurance phases? Have you felt the discomfort in the weight room? Is there any particular exercise that causes the discomfort? If so, eliminate that exercise or replace it with one that doesn't cause discomfort. Be especially cautious with the squat. Also, be sure to use a platform for the step-up that is not higher than midshin. Be careful with the leg press during the Power Endurance phase. Pushing the platform up so explosively that it leaves your feet, only to slam back down on fully extended and locked knees can cause cartilage damage.
- Have you recently changed your bike setup? The most common cause in this category is lowering or raising the

saddle too much, too soon. Small, incremental changes of perhaps a quarter-inch per week are recommended. Do you have new pedals? Are they adjusted properly? A bike shop can help with this. Have you changed cleat position?

- Have you recently fallen or crashed?
- Are you getting adequate protein and iron in your diet? Low intakes of these nutrients have been associated with injury. Chapter 9 covers the details of diet selection.

For most injuries common to cycling, initial treatment usually involves rest, icing, compression, and elevation. The acronym RICE may help you remember this standard therapy. Rest the injured site by not using it. Apply an ice compact for about 15 minutes once an hour, with a cloth between the skin and the ice to prevent frostbite. A bag of frozen peas is perfect for most injuries because it conforms well to the area. Just don't eat the peas after several thaw-refreezing cycles. A light compress such as an Ace bandage wrap may also help to immobilize the area and prevent swelling and further discomfort.

If forced to reduce riding during an injury, you can maintain cardiovascular endurance, and you can stay sane, by cross-training. The best activities for injured cyclists include Nordic skiing, swimming, stair-climbing machines, walking, and in-line skating.

Osteoarthritis

Anyone who has been on this earth for a half century or more has some osteoarthritis, although it may have no measurable impact on riding or daily activities. Those who have it badly enough know how debilitating osteoarthritis is. Cycling is usually one activity that can continue despite the condition.

The pain of osteoarthritis results from thinning cartilage on the ends of bones at the joints. In advanced stages, the cartilage covers are completely worn away and the bones touch. Without any cushioning or lubrication, limited movement and pain result. Afflicted joints that commonly affect cycling are wrists, elbows, and, especially, knees.

The causes of osteoarthritis are not known, but three are

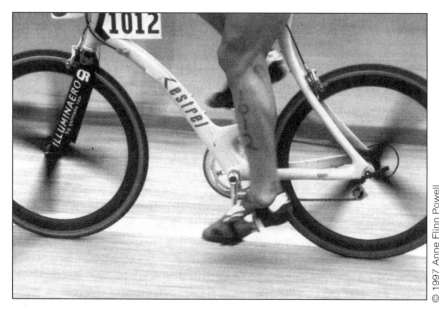

The downsides from living a half-century are the aches and pains.

suspected. Heredity is one. Several generations of a family are frequently inflicted. Another possible cause is an injury that occurred earlier in life and damaged the cartilage. In the same category is surgery to remove cartilage, as was done 20 or more years ago. Most of these surgeries resulted from extrinsic injuries suffered in contact sports such as football. Historically, athletic participation was thought to be a cause of osteoarthritis. However, in recent years, numerous studies of sports ranging from running to soccer to parachuting have found no connection between athletics and osteoarthritis. In fact, other studies have shown that load-bearing activities, such as cycling, actually decrease the ailment's incidence. On the other hand, one long-term study found that the most active subjects, as well as obese subjects, were at the greatest risk for osteoarthritis. The jury is still out on the cause.

Riding with osteoarthritis is largely a matter of discovering what conditions make it worse and how to care for your joints when it flares up. One of the worst conditions for arthritic joints is riding in cold weather. A long warm-up may help, as may wearing warm clothing, especially around the joints. A neoprene sheath, available in many drug stores, may help on these days.

Common self-treatment includes using nonsteroidal anti-inflammatories such as aspirin and ibuprofen. Be conservative with their use, however, as common side effects from long-term use include stomach irritation and intestinal bleeding. Ibuprofen is likely to have a less negative effect on your gut. Your doctor may inject a corticosteroid into the joint to reduce inflammation. This is typically not done more than three times for any joint. A promising self-treatment uses glucosamine sulfate (see sidebar).

More than likely, you can continue riding even if osteoarthritis symptoms appear. Riding may help relieve the problems by strengthening the cartilage, bringing in nutrients, and removing waste products.

TREATING TWINGES IN THE HINGES

Joint pain that accompanies aging can interfere with riding—especially when it shows up in the knees. Until now there has been little you could do about it except cut back on saddle time. This condition is known as osteoarthritis and is marked by pain due to wearing away joint cartilage. For years, osteoarthritis has been treated in the United States with nonsteroidal anti-inflammatory drugs such as aspirin and ibuprofen. These drugs relieve the symptoms but do little or nothing to reverse the condition. Now a compound that has been used on animals in this country and has become popular in Europe is raising hope for those who suffer from osteoarthritis. The compound is *glucosamine sulfate.*

Several worldwide studies conducted on glucosamine sulfate have found that it relieves the symptoms of osteoarthritis in all joints and appears to reverse joint damage by fortifying cartilage. It is nontoxic, being found naturally in small amounts in many foods, is safe for long-term use, and has no known reactions to other drugs. In one study, the chief complaint of some subjects who were treated with glucosamine sulfate was heartburn. It's more gentle on the body than aspirin.

When taken orally, it is rapidly absorbed by the tissues and quickly works to rebuild damaged cartilage, a rubbery cover on the ends of bones. Improvement is apparent after as little as two weeks of daily dosage, with cartilage substantially rebuilt after 30 days of treatment. Improvement seems to last for 6 to 12 weeks after ending treatment, indicating a need to take it periodically.

Glucosamine sulfate is effective for early and mild cases of osteoarthritis and less helpful for severe symptoms when there is little or no cartilage left in the joint. It has even been shown effective in treating chondromalacia patella, another knee injury common in cyclists.

As a natural product, glucosamine sulfate is not patentable, so don't expect U.S. drug companies to start making it. Instead, it is produced and marketed by nutritional supplement companies and sold through health food stores. Although expensive as supplements go, it typically sells for about $30 for a one-month supply of capsules. Alternately using glucosamine sulfate for six to eight weeks, then stopping it for the same number of weeks effectively reduces the long-term cost. A daily dosage of 1,500 milligrams, divided into two or three doses, was the standard intake in most clinical studies. Higher doses appear safe but may not provide any greater benefits.

Before starting glucosamine sulfate, it's a good idea to talk with your health care provider.

9

Fueling

"You are what you eat." How many times have you heard that old saw? Probably hundreds, if not thousands, of times. Have you ever paused to think about what it really means? Consider, for example, that the food you eat provides the building blocks for the ongoing maintenance and replacement of cells. The energy from food, in the form of sugar and fat, restocks depot sites in your muscles, adipose tissues, blood, and liver. Nutrients in the food you eat keep bodily systems, such as the immune system, functioning. Food is also critical for repairing cells damaged during intense and long rides. You definitely are what you eat.

Age appears to play a role in making food choices. With rare exceptions, young cyclists think about quantity of food, and what's in that food is of little consequence. However, youth is a powerful aid in correcting mistakes made in dietary selection. Successful aging riders know that it is the quality of food that matters most. For the past-50 cyclist, there is little room for error in any aspect of training, especially diet.

Some aging riders take wholesome foods for granted, yet look for a dietary supplement, the magic pill, that will bring peak performance. There are many promising ergogenic aids on the market, some of which boost riding strength and endurance, but none are as powerful as a nutrient-dense diet.

In the last 20 years, sports nutritionists have learned a great deal about food as fuel, but theirs is still a young science. Much remains to be learned, especially as it relates to a given rider's unique needs. We know next to nothing about how diet affects endurance cyclists past the half-century mark. Science does know, however, that individuals can respond to a given diet in unique ways. For example, some cannot tolerate dairy products. Others have no trouble with dairy but don't digest wheat products well. It's also known that a diet high in cholesterol puts some at risk for heart disease, but for others it presents no problem. Such gross examples point out that genetics plays a role in dietary selection, so there is not a single diet that works for every rider. Your experience counts for a lot.

The purpose of this chapter is to explore some recent trends in sports nutrition. You should also read the many books and stories in cycling magazines that discuss a more traditional position on the athlete's diet. From the many possibilities, adopt what works for your unique needs as a past-50 cyclist. Let's begin by brushing up on the basics of sports nutrition.

Energy for Endurance

Whether it's a carrot or a sports drink, food is merely stored energy derived from the sun. The chemical bonds that hold the carrot or sports drink together are easily broken down by the human digestive system, altering the energy into a form that meets the immediate needs of the working muscles or is stored for later use. Food is divided into three categories—fat, carbohydrate, and protein. Each has unique characteristics that benefit cycling. Each also has disadvantages.

Fat

In the last 20 years American society has come to think of dietary fat as the enemy. We vilify and avoid it at every opportunity. The marketing of food now capitalizes on fat phobia by advertising products as low fat or, better yet, fat free. What's the source of this fear? Why after eons of fat consumption by our ancestors, and even by most of us before the 1970s, have we recently come to believe that all fat is bad? It goes back to a Boston University study that began in 1948 and continues to this day. Researchers enlisted the 28,000 residents of the small town of Framingham, Massachusetts, to be studied the rest of their lives.

What initially came from the Framingham study was a set of risk factors for heart disease, which was and still is the leading cause of death among Americans. One of these initially apparent risk factors was a diet high in cholesterol and saturated fat. Starting in the 1960s, public service announcements, newspaper articles, books, and talk shows made this risk factor familiar to most of us. Fat was getting a bad reputation.

Indeed, other studies have supported the Framingham contention that the saturated fats found mainly in animal products, such as meat and dairy, may lead to heart disease in some people. Saturated fat, however, does not represent all fat. The other major divisions of the fat family are called

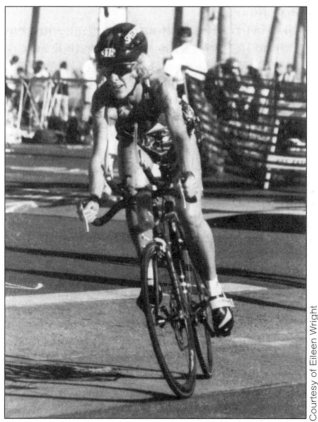

54-year old Eileen Wright at the Imperial Beach Duathlon, 1997.

polyunsaturated and monounsaturated fats. Polyunsaturated fats are found mostly in vegetable oils. Monounsaturated fats are present in such foods as nuts, avocado, and olive oil. A relative newcomer to the fat family is a manufactured product called hydrogenated fat. This is a polyunsaturated fat that has been chemically altered to give it the same characteristics as saturated fat. It's found in margarine and many snack foods.

Of the unsaturated fats, some polyunsaturated fats have been associated with an increased risk of heart disease and even cancer when eaten in large amounts. The other real villain for heart disease, besides some types of saturated fat, is hydrogenated fat. Partially hydrogenated vegetable oil increases the blood levels of LDL cholesterol (bad cholesterol) much as saturated fat does. Unlike saturated fat, it also lowers levels of HDL cholesterol (good cholesterol), making it a double whammy for the heart.

Based on most research, it appears that you should probably limit some fats, such as hydrogenated, saturated, and polyunsaturated vegetable oils, in your diet. Don't take that to mean all fats, however. Some are good for your health and performance. Take the oils found in deep-water fish, for example. Two polyunsaturated fats, eicosapentaenoic acid (EPA) and docosahexenoic acid (DHA), in such fish as tuna, herring, sardines, and mackerel, lower the risk of heart disease. You may also see these referred to as omega-3 fats. Monounsaturated fats provide similar benefits.

Research on the effect of fat on disease and performance continues. A 1996 study at the State University of New York challenges the idea that dietary fat is a heart disease risk factor for athletes. In this 12-week study, 12 male and 13 female runners, who ran at least 35 miles per week, ate either a low-fat diet with 16 percent of calories from fat, or a high-fat diet with either 30 percent or 42 percent of calories from fat. On both high-fat diets, saturated fat made up about a third of the total fat consumed, or about 10 to 15 percent of daily calories. Cholesterol intake on the high-fat diets increased by 40 to 56 percent. After four weeks on each diet, the risk factors associated with heart disease were significantly reduced on the high-fat diets when compared with the low-fat diet. This included, on the high-fat diet, an increased HDL-cholesterol count and lower triglyceride levels. The subjects also maintained their body weights, percent body fat, and blood pressures on the high-fat diets. This means that eating a high-fat diet was beneficial in terms of risk for heart disease in these athletes. Another way to look at it is that the low-fat diet increased the risk of heart disease. It is unclear if these changes would occur over longer periods than 12 weeks or in sedentary people.

Fat stored in the body plays a major role in cycling performance. The average, lean 150-pound rider has stored about 94,000 calories in fat. That's enough energy to ride at a moderate effort from New York City to Salt Lake City. For comparison, the energy socked away as carbohydrate in the same rider would fuel a trip from New York City to Poughkeepsie, NY—about 50 miles.

Even in the skinniest rider there are huge quantities of energy available in fat. The problem is accessing it. The sedentary person's body preferentially chooses carbohydrate for fuel during activity, which explains, at least in part, why the endurance of out-of-shape people is poor. With more time spent on the bike, the amount of fat you burn relative to carbohydrate increases. That's one reason the Base period of training emphasizes low intensity and high volume.

Recent studies have demonstrated that eating a diet with a moderately high amount of fat improves the ability to use stored fat as fuel, while sparing the body's limited levels of carbohydrate. On a high-carbohydrate, low-fat diet, carbohydrate is slightly preferred by the working muscles.

Carbohydrate

There is no doubt that carbohydrate is critical to endurance performance on a bike. In college physiology classes, instructors are fond of pointing out to students that "fat burns in a carbohydrate flame." What this means is that, although you may burn little carbohydrate as fuel during a workout, if carbohydrate is depleted, fat burning proceeds with more difficulty, and so the workout is done. Cyclists call this phenomenon the bonk.

As pointed out earlier, there's not much carbohydrate socked away in the body of the average cyclist. About 1,500 to 2,000 calories, enough for two to two-and-a-half hours of moderately intense riding, is stored in the body, with 75 percent of this in the muscles and most of the remainder in the liver. A small amount, about 1 percent, is floating around in the blood.

During the first 10 minutes of a ride, carbohydrate metabolism increases rapidly, then more gradually. When the intensity of the ride goes up, as in climbing a hill or doing intervals, the percentage of carbohydrate you use to fuel the ride goes up also. During an intense ride at well above lactate threshold, carbohydrate may provide nearly all the required energy, rapidly depleting the available stores. For long or hard rides, replacing this fuel source with a sports drink or food is critical to continuing.

Fortunately, meeting carbohydrate needs is easy. Grocery stores are bursting at the seams with foodstuffs high in carbohydrate. Unfortunately, much of it is best left on the shelves, but more on that later. For some reason, cyclists think of grains as being the best, if not the only, source of carbohydrate available in the market. They're not. Also high in carbohydrate are vegetables and fruits, which are much more nutrient dense than grains and have nutrients that are more absorbable. Grains, such as wheat or oats, are inedible grass seeds in their raw state and must go through a lengthy process of husking, grinding, mixing, and heating to produce consumable foods such as bread and cereal. These grain-based foods are called starches. A diet high in starchy foods has unique health and performance consequences.

Carbohydrates are a form of sugar. Three of the most common sugar components of carbohydrates are sucrose, glucose, and fructose. Sucrose is found in table sugar, glucose makes up starches, and fructose is the sugar in some fruits. These sugars go different routes once in the body before providing energy to turn the cranks. Sucrose is broken down during digestion into glucose and fructose. Fructose is sent to the liver where it is converted into glucose, delaying the release of energy. Glucose provides energy the fastest, as it goes directly into the bloodstream from the small intestine. In 1981, scientists began classifying foods containing types and amounts of sugars based on how quickly they get from the mouth to the muscles. The system they developed is called the glycemic index. Foods high on the glycemic index are rapidly absorbed,

GLYCEMIC INDEX OF COMMON FOODS

High glycemic index (80% or higher)

Bread, French	Corn flakes	Corn Chex	Crispix	Grapenuts Flakes
Molasses	Parsnips	Pasta, rice	Potatoes, baked	Potatoes, instant
Rice cakes	Rice Chex	Rice, instant	Rice Krispies	Rice, white
Tapioca	Tofu frozen dessert			

Moderate glycemic index (50%-80%)

All-Bran cereal	Apricots	Bagels	Bananas	Barley
Beets	Black bean soup	Bread, pita	Bread, rye	Bread, wheat
Bread, white	Corn chips	Cornmeal	Corn, sweet	Couscous
Crackers	Doughnuts	Ice cream	Mango	Muesli
Muffins	Oat bran	Oatmeal	Orange juice	Pea soup
Pineapple	Popcorn	Potato chips	Potatoes, boiled	Potatoes, mashed
Potatoes, sweet	PowerBar	Pumpkin	Raisins	Rice, brown
Rye crisps	Soft drinks	Taco shells	Watermelon	Yams

Low glycemic index (30%-50%)

Yogurt, fruit	Apple	Apple juice	Apple sauce	Beans, baked
Beans, black	Beans, lima	Beans, pinto	Chocolate	Grapefruit juice
Grapes	Kiwifruit	Oranges	Pasta	Pears
Peas, black-eyed	Peas, split	Rye	Tomato soup	

Very low glycemic index (less than 30%)

Barley	Beans, kidney	Beans, soy	Cherries	Grapefruit
Lentils	Milk	Peaches	Peanuts	Plums

From Foster-Powell, K., and J.B. Miller. 1995. International tables of glycemic index. *American Journal of Clinical Nutrition* 62: 871S-893S. © Am. J. Clin. Nutr. American Society for Clinical Nutrition. Adapted by permission.

and low-glycemic index foods release their energy slowly. Table 9.1 classifies common foods as high, moderate, low, or very low glycemic.

The concept of glycemic index is important for riders in two ways. During and immediately after a ride, the muscles' demand for fuel, especially carbohydrate, is great. This demand is quickly met by high-glycemic index foods. Once outside the time when rapid replacement of energy is a priority, eating low-glycemic index foods moderates the swings in blood sugar. Eating moderate- to high-glycemic index foods is usually accompanied by a frequent feeling of hunger. Consuming foods low on the glycemic index is beneficial in other ways, too. Low-glycemic index foods are associated with less body fat, because excess sugar in the blood is stored as fat. Eating low-glycemic index foods throughout most of the day also means a lowered risk for heart disease, because excess blood sugars elevate triglycerides, which lower HDL (good cholesterol) production. When low-glycemic index foods make up the bulk of the carbohydrates you eat, you reduce the risk for adult-onset diabetes, which is common in Americans beyond the age of 40.

It's interesting to note that the rise of heart disease as a cause of death in this country has paralleled the consumption of sugar. Figure 9.1 shows that sugar in the American diet has increased from 63 pounds per person in 1895 to 140 pounds for each of us annually almost a century later. The greatest increase in sugar consumption in the last decade is due to using high fructose corn syrup (HFCS) as a sweetener in such foods as soft drinks, catsup, baked goods, canned fruits, most sports drinks, and energy bars. In 1980, each American, on average, ate 19 pounds of HFCS. By 1994 we were eating 56 pounds annually, nearly three times as much. HFCS is a corn starch chemically converted to fructose to make it taste sweeter. It's about half glucose and half fructose.

Starch makes up about 50 percent of the average American's carbohydrate intake, with most of the remainder coming about evenly from sucrose and HFCS. There's no reason to believe that cyclists don't also eat such a diet, and perhaps consume even more sugar than the average. Besides the already mentioned health risks that sugar poses, there is also empirical evidence that a diet high in sugars weakens the immune

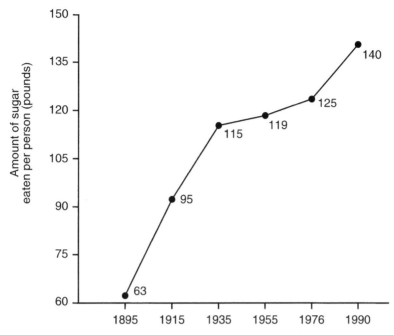

Figure 9.1 Annual sugar consumption in the American diet, 1895 to 1990
Excerpted from "What are Americans Eating?" in Jan/Feb issue of *Nutrition Alert*,
4742 Liberty Road, S, Suite 148; Salem, OR 97302.

system. This is of particular concern to riders who are frequently run down and ill, especially when they increase the workload of training.

Protein

In the 1800s athletes and physicians believed that protein was the primary fuel for physical activity. In the early 20th century, however, scientists discovered that fat and carbohydrate provide the energy for exercise. This information was not well disseminated, so from the time of World War II through the Vietnam War era, American cyclists were still being advised to eat a diet high in protein. In the 1970s, scientific studies on the role of carbohydrate were so well publicized by the popular media that diets began to change. In the scientific literature, little interest was shown in the role of protein. As a result, the current recommended dietary allowance (RDA) for protein does not account for the impact of physical training levels on dietary needs.

Since the early 1980s, high-carbohydrate eating has been in fashion, especially for athletes, and protein consumption has been greatly reduced by many cyclists. We have a tendency to overcorrect in our society, often requiring decades for the pendulum to swing back the other way. Such a shifting of opinions is now occurring on the subject of protein consumption, especially by endurance athletes.

In our rush to embrace the scientific wisdom of the last few decades with its advice to avoid the cholesterol and the fat of meat, we forgot that protein is an essential component of the dietary needs of cyclists. We threw out the baby with the bath water. More recent research indicates that by eating too little

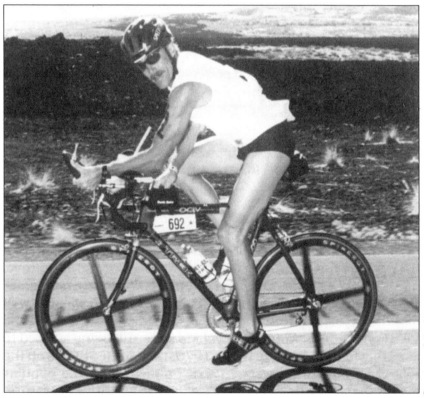

Jim Hunter eating on the move at the Hawaii Ironman, 1997.

Courtesy of Jim Hunter

protein, a rider compromises health while undermining training and performance. Without adequate protein, the cyclist's body is missing its only source of amino acids to make new proteins for hormones, enzymes, immune system cells, and oxygen-carrying hemoglobin.

For a cyclist who weighs more than 130 pounds and is training with high volume and frequent, intense rides, the RDA of 50 to 65 grams of protein is woefully inadequate. For bigger riders on such a diet, muscle wasting, loss of strength, long recoveries from workouts, and frequent illness are likely. For the past-50 cyclist, the need for protein is even greater. Studies suggest that with aging, protein is poorly digested and absorbed. The losses in lean body mass and the common illnesses usually associated with aging may be due in part to inadequate protein in the diet.

The RDA for protein was determined using sedentary people and is probably still adequate for their needs. When riding intensely or for long distances, however, the body uses some protein for fuel as carbohydrate stores are depleted. Strength training places an even greater demand on the system for protein. The primary storage sites for protein are muscle. Hard riding and strength training combined with low protein intake can easily result in the body cannibalizing itself to provide energy. The best way to avoid this scenario is by eating protein, especially from meat because its protein is better absorbed than that from vegetable sources.

The best source of meat is wild game because these animals are lower in saturated fat and have about one-seventh the total fat of corn-fed, feedlot cattle. However, unless you hunt or have a local store that sells wild game, this is not practical. The next best choice is the meats of open range-fed or organically raised cattle. The fat content of such animals is similar to wild game. Both types are also high in the heart-healthy omega-3 fats discussed earlier, and low in omega-6 fats. In addition, wild and organic meat doesn't have any chemical residues from antibiotics or growth hormones as feedlot meat often has.

How much protein do you need? Recent studies on young athletes suggest that a cyclist needs .5 to .7 grams of protein per pound of body weight. Although there are no studies on aging athletes, an over-50 cyclist may need .1 to .2 grams per pound more. Assuming a need for .6 to .9 grams per pound, a 150-pound, 50-year-old rider would eat 90 to 135 grams of protein daily while training hard. How much is that? Table 9.2 lists the protein content of some common foods.

Table 9.2

PROTEIN CONTENT (IN GRAMS) OF COMMON FOODS

Food	Protein content (g)
Dairy	
Milk, 8 oz	8
Yogurt, 1 c	12
Cheese, 1 oz	8
Cottage cheese, 1 c	24
Ice cream, 1 c	4
Vegetables	
Kidney beans, 1/2 c	7
Pinto beans, 1/2 c	6
Black beans, 1/2 c	8
Tomato, 1/2 c	1
Beets, 1/2 c	1
Broccoli, 2 spears	3
Peas, 2/3 c	4
Lentils, 1 c	15.5
Soybeans, 1 c	20
Tofu, 4 oz	8.5
Meats	
Tuna fish, 2 oz	15
Salmon, 2 oz	11
Chicken, 1/2 breast	30
Ground beef, 4 oz	20
Pork chops, 1/4 lb	16
Turkey, 4 oz	10
Scallops, 3 oz	14
Other	
Walnuts, 12	7
Bread, 1 slice	3
Tortilla, 1	6

Can you eat too much protein? Textbooks often discuss the hazards of eating a diet high in protein, but the potential downside is exaggerated. For example, kidney problems are often cited but are based on studies done on sedentary people with impaired kidney function. It is important, however, to drink lots of water when protein makes up a substantial portion of your diet because water losses are increased. The possibility of dehydration is increased as protein intake rises, because body fluids are used to urinate away the by-products of protein metabolism.

What should you eat? The answer to that question has changed over the years and will likely continue to change. In the 1940s, cyclists were advised to eat a diet high in green vegetables and meat and to avoid starchy foods such as white bread and potatoes. By the end of the 1980s, the dietary advice for riders had shifted 180 degrees: Eat more carbohydrates, especially complex carbohydrates such as breads and pasta, and less meat. Now there is an undercurrent of change taking place among athletes and scientists. Some question the current recommendations and urge a return to a diet closer to that of the 1940s.

What you should eat is probably different from what your training partner should eat. We're each different. Some cannot digest the sugars in milk, and others seem to thrive on it. Wheat presents problems for some, but not others. These are only gross maladaptations that we can easily observe. There are undoubtedly minor maladaptations that aren't as obvious and have a more sinister affect on health and performance. No one can tell you exactly what these may be because the science of nutrition is still young, and little or no research has been done on individualizing nutrition.

The safest diet, and one that is likely to benefit cycling performance, includes plenty of lean meat, fish, poultry, and shellfish, and all the fruits and vegetables you can comfortably eat. Such a diet includes small amounts of nuts and dried fruits as snacks, greatly limiting high- and moderate-glycemic index carbohydrates, processed foods, vegetable oils, and hydrogenated fats. Except during and immediately following a workout, sugar is best avoided.

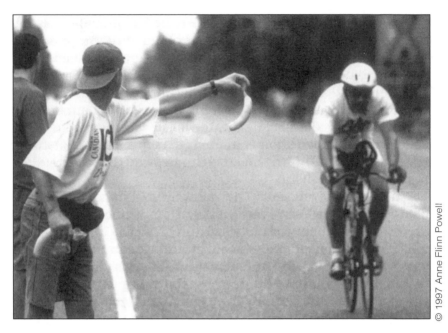

The banana vs. the rider. Fueling up makes the rider a winner all around.

© 1997 Anne Flinn Powell

Vegetarianism

Past-50 cyclists often adopt a vegetarian diet in the belief that it will improve performance by making them leaner and healthier. Switching to a strict diet devoid of animal products is more likely to result in deteriorating cycling performance. The more restrictive a diet is, the greater the possibility that some nutrient deficiency will limit normal physiological function.

Vegetarians, especially vegans who eat no animal-based foods, are typically low in essential amino acids and fats, and in calcium, iron, zinc, phosphorous, and vitamins A, B12, and D. Although all these present problems for the serious cyclist, iron deficiency is particularly worrisome. Low iron levels are associated with poor endurance, low power, high risk of injury, and mental depression. Getting adequate iron in the diet is necessary for continued improvement on the bike. Vegan diets complicate this need. Only about 2 to 10 percent of iron from plant sources is absorbed by the body, whereas 10 to 25 percent of animal iron is taken up. Even iron supplements aren't as readily absorbed as the iron in meat. If you're a vegan who drinks tea or coffee with meals, or if you eat a lot of whole-grain foods, you further reduce iron absorption from plant sources.

Studies have shown that vegetarian athletes are typically low in sex hormones. Diminished levels of testosterone in men and estrogen in women means longer recovery following hard workouts. These growth hormones are necessary for muscle repair.

If you decide to follow a vegetarian diet, educating yourself about nutrition is intrinsic to success on the bike, or you may experience diminished performance. One way to resolve this problem is to eat dairy products and eggs regularly in your meals, as they include adequate amounts of the nutrients lacking in a vegan diet. You may also want to talk with your doctor about supplementing with creatine, a chemical found in muscle tissue, which the body uses to produce creatine phosphate, a high-octane fuel used for brief, but powerful muscle contractions.

10

Psyching

Who would have believed it? Just 28 months before, Greg LeMond was lying in a pool of blood in a California woods, the casualty of a fluke hunting accident. Now he was standing on the victory platform of the world's greatest bicycle race—the Tour de France. Many had predicted the shotgun blast would end his career. After all, a collapsed lung with a section missing, the loss of three-fourths of his blood supply, two broken ribs, pellets lodged in his heart and other vital organs, and hovering on the verge of death for several hours had to have serious implications for professional cycling. Then, of course, there was the atrophy that came from lying around during the long recovery. Eight weeks following the accident he was 20 pounds lighter, the result of muscle loss, and he was 18-percent body fat. Hardly the stuff of Tour de France victories.

Yet, somehow, LeMond overcame the physical disabilities. More important, he overcame the self-doubt that plagued him for the next year to take the victory—and in a spectacular way.

The final stage of the 1989 Tour was a flat, downhill 24.5-kilometer time trial from Versailles to the Arc de Triomphe on the Champs-Elysees in Paris. Coming into this stage, LeMond had surprised everyone by holding onto second place in his first Tour since a win in 1986. Standing in the starter's gate on the last day of the race, he was only 50 seconds behind Frenchman Laurent Fignon. But 50 seconds may as well be forever with only one short stage remaining. Even his most ardent supporters knew it would take a miracle to make up 50 ticks of the clock in 15.24 miles. They were proud and happy that he had fought his way back from a devastating injury and come so close to victory. What more could they have expected?

LeMond didn't share their satisfaction. "I want it all. I really want to win this race," he told a reporter before the last stage. "I'm convinced that it's still possible." Before starting, he instructed the crew in his support car not to give him time checks along the course, as is customary. He wanted nothing to break his concentration. This would be nothing short of an all-out effort.

"I didn't think; I just rode," LeMond would say later. And ride he did—35.95 miles per hour, the fastest any man had ever gone in the history of the Tour de France. Starting second from last, he now had to wait at the finish line to see if Fignon could match or even come close to his time. All the Frenchman had to do was post a time 49 seconds slower and the yellow jersey was his to keep.

Five kilometers into the race, Fignon was told he was already six seconds down, and he briefly stopped pedaling as he looked back over his shoulder in disbelief. After 11.5 kilometers, Fignon was down by 21 seconds. At 14 kilometers he was trailing by 24 seconds. After 18 kilometers there was a 35-second deficit, after 20 kilometers, 45 seconds. "All I could think of was how terrible it would be to lose by one second," LeMond remembered thinking at this point. With 50 meters to go the clock showed that Fignon was now down 50 seconds. Greg LeMond had won.

It was the smallest margin of victory in the Tour's history. A mere eight seconds separated them after 3,285 kilometers of racing. Greg LeMond was back on the victory platform of the Tour de France for the second time. It was an unlikely ending to what had appeared a tragedy just a few months before.

You Gotta Believe

LeMond could have accepted second place, yet still ridden hard. Practically no one believed it was possible to make up 50 seconds that day, especially because he had been through such a harrowing ordeal in the previous two years. That he was able to pull it off is usually credited to his use of aerodynamic, triathlon handlebars. The real reason was because LeMond wanted it badly and believed he could do it.

Possibly the most important psychological skill for success in cycling, as in any aspect of life, is believing in yourself. "If you think you can or you think you can't, you're probably right," Henry Ford is supposed to have said. Greg LeMond thought he could, and he did. It's easy to find excuses, or reasons, why something is outside our realm of possibilities. The most common reason used is age. "I'm too old," is another way of saying, "I don't believe I can, and age is the best excuse I can find." Riders in their 80s and 90s compete on the track and roads, complete century rides, ride coast to coast, and accomplish more than most Americans in their 30s. They don't use age as an excuse; they use it as a reason to keep going. They believe in themselves. You can, too.

DO YOU BELIEVE?

There is more to cycling success than being fit. The mental aspects of competition are every bit as important, if not more so.

Perhaps the most important and basic mental skill is believing in yourself. Weakness in this area undermines your efforts to improve by eroding self-esteem and magnifying obstacles. Riders with low confidence find that just showing up for a race or century ride takes great courage. Poor performance is practically assured.

Do you believe in yourself? Let's explore your cycling confidence with the following attitude survey. Respond to each statement honestly, as if no one else will see the resulting profile.

Scoring System

| 1 Never | 2 Seldom | 3 Sometimes | 4 Usually | 5 Always |

___ 1. I believe my potential as a cyclist is excellent.

___ 2. I think of myself more as a success than as a failure.

___ 3. I'm able to train and perform at near my ability level.

___ 4. People see me as a tough competitor.

___ 5. In cycling events I am mentally tough.

___ 6. My confidence stays high in the days after a poor performance.

___ 7. Before events, I am sure I will do well.

___ 8. I can take risks during an event without fear of failure.

___ 9. Adverse weather conditions give me a psychological advantage.

___ 10. I perform well in events regardless of who shows up.

Now add the answers you gave and compare the total with the following standards.

Score Profile

45-50 You have excellent confidence and can perform well if your training and diet are sound.

40-44 You're a solid performer, but have occasional lapses. Fine tuning your mental skills will make you more consistent.

35-39 If your training and diet are sound, you may be riding well most of the time. If they aren't, you're riding well below your potential.

27-34 You are probably inconsistent in training, and it shows in your events as well. When your body and mind are both performing optimally, you ride well.

10-26 You probably see little relationship between what you think and how you ride. You may believe that you just weren't given what it takes to do well. You must read and study to improve your confidence before you'll improve your riding.

You can enhance your belief in yourself by learning more about applied sport psychology. Other than this book, reading others such as those listed in the references section at the end of the book will help.

To get the most from yourself, not just in cycling but in all of life's endeavors, set challenging goals that you believe are achievable regardless of your age. Without that belief, all the fancy equipment and scientific training in the world won't work. You've got to believe.

Mental Training

Learning to believe in yourself is a form of mental fitness and can be trained, just as you've learned to train for physical fitness. It's something that you do every day, on and off the bike. To get in shape mentally, you must develop and constantly hone three skills:

- Positive attitude
- High motivation to excel
- Great pride in accomplishments

Positive Attitude

Every day you are bombarded with feedback about your worth as an individual and as a cyclist. Some of this comes from others as a comment or more subtly through facial expression or body language. Most of it, however, is internal and never heard by anyone else. What you say to yourself is more powerful than what others say about you. The little voice in your head can be your strongest ally or your greatest enemy. You decide which.

Only you can control what the little voice says. If you've trained it to find fault and point out shortcomings, you will seldom achieve success. If, on the other hand, your self-talk is positive, attaining peak performance on the bike is practically assured. Negative self-talk focuses your mind on the obstacles. A positive attitude allows you to clearly see beyond the obstacles to the possibilities for goal attainment.

Eliminate the "what ifs" and focus on the challenge at hand. Oh, sure there will still be setbacks. That's the way life is. Instead of dwelling on what you could have done, look for the learning experience in every misfortune. The only difference between winning and losing is that when we lose, we learn something. Eliminate the negatives and replace them with positives.

Imagine how boring and unfulfilling life would be without obstacles. Where would the thrill of victory come from if there wasn't an agony of defeat? Obstacles are good. Accept them while focusing on their challenges and you will enjoy satisfaction and fulfillment in life. Wallow in them and you assure defeat. Some opposition is necessary for attainment. Kites rise against, not with, the wind.

Defeat, in whatever form, is often blamed on physical obstacles, such as lack of endurance, strength, or speed. The negative thinker sees this as insurmountable. The cyclist with a positive attitude instead sees two opportunities. One opportunity involves taking advantage of known strengths. For example, if speed is lacking but endurance is good, the smart racer will keep the average speed high in the closing miles of a race to take the speed out of the sprinters' legs. The other opportunity is to improve weaknesses. That means concentrating a good portion of training time on the limiter that is holding you back the most. Endurance, strength, and speed can all be improved.

The most incredible machine in the world is the human body. With all that science has learned about anatomy, biology, physiology, and biomechanics in the last 500 years, we are still far from fully understanding how it works. New discoveries are made almost daily, yet there is more that remains unknown than known. Science does know that, contrary to what happens to machines, the human machine gets better the more it's used.

No two people are exactly alike. Uniqueness is a characteristic of human physiology. You have the only body like yours

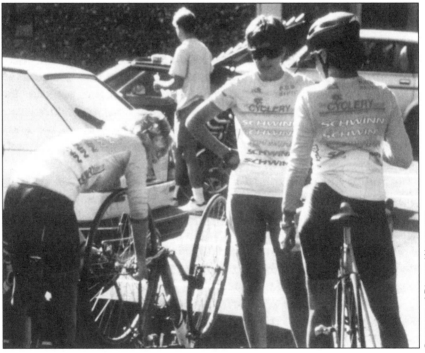

Courtesy of Dianna Waggoner

Parking lot, pre-race preparation and chat.

in the universe. Learn to listen to what it tells you every day through subtle sensations and responses to training. Develop it to its fullest by seeing and reinforcing the possibilities every day.

What can you do if you don't see the possibilities, if instead you are continually reinforcing the negatives every day? First, recognizing shortcomings and willingness to change is 90 percent of developing a positive attitude. The final 10 percent comes with positive reinforcement practiced daily. Here's a strategy that will help. Every night when you go to bed, between the time when the lights go out and falling asleep, review in your mind the successes of the day, no matter how small they were. Perhaps you completed a workout that was difficult. Revel in its accomplishment one more time. Maybe you climbed that hill locals call "The Wall" better than you have before. Relive the accomplishment. It could even be something as seemingly minor as getting on your bike when motivation was low. Remember and relive your successes every day, and your attitude and belief in yourself will improve dramatically.

High Motivation

In the final analysis, it's really not high-tech training, the latest equipment, or a perfect diet that make you a successful cyclist. Motivation is the key. A burning desire to succeed makes the difference. Motivation is what gets you on the bike on a cold, gray day. Motivation also gets you into bed just as a great show is starting on television. Remember the old saying, "As you sow, so shall you reap." It's true: You get nothing for nothing. There is a price to pay for success.

The path to top performance on a bike, as in any endeavor in life, is not crowded. Accomplishment in cycling takes a lot of effort and sacrifice. Too much for most, even for those who have natural ability. There are people walking around the streets of every city who were born to excel in some sport such as cycling. Genetically and physiologically they were given the stuff of champions. These naturally gifted were physically programmed to win the Tour de France, to break the hour record, to succeed as no one before, not even the great Eddie Merck, has done. However, today they lead mundane lives following a standard routine, never knowing they were the chosen. They've wasted the talent by letting circumstances lead them down the easy path. They're skating through life with little challenge or fulfillment.

You may not have been born to win the Tour, but are you wasting your talent? Are you letting life take the lead, or are you in control of your destiny? Pursue excellence every day. Attack life and get all you can from it. Stay on the lookout for new ideas. Seek new ways to excel. Life is too short to do otherwise.

All that you have accomplished so far in life resulted from lots of blood, sweat, and tears. It's the same with cycling. You've weathered the storms, literally and figuratively, to improve fitness. You love the sport. Wouldn't it be dumb to put in all that time and effort, then not expect the best of yourself? The time to begin is now—not tomorrow or the next day. Every moment that slips through your fingers without doing your best is time lost, time you can never get back again.

Pride in Accomplishments

Most Americans, especially those in our generation, were taught to play down, to devalue, personal accomplishment. In the same manner, we learned that love of self is a cardinal sin and leads to arrogance, conceit, and snobbery that diminishes the value of others. Our teachers were well meaning, but this way of thinking encourages failure. Until this schooled attitude is replaced with respect for self and a healthy pride in personal accomplishments, attainment of exceptionally high goals is not possible in cycling or any other endeavor of life.

Your self-esteem determines how you behave. For example, nothing affects the ability to get along with others as much as the image you hold of yourself. Constantly put yourself down, and others will think less of you also. Love yourself, and you're capable of loving others and being loved. The same goes for cycling. Belittle what you've accomplished, and others will adopt that attitude, setting up a negative feedback loop. Take pride in your accomplishments, and others will also hold them in high esteem, reinforcing your value as a person and as a cyclist.

Be careful, though, as pride has a narrow edge. On one side is self-respect and a healthy pleasure that comes from achievement. On the other is the egocentric and prima donna attitude that turns others away. You must honor what you've achieved without boastfulness. Quiet and inward pride is the key. How can you do that? The following are five characteristics of a healthy attitude based on the acronym PRIDE.

P Is for Perseverance

Nothing worth having in cycling, as in life, comes easily. It's the hard challenges, the steep climbs and long rides, we face that bring pride. Don't avoid them; rather seek them out. Though hard, any reasonable goal is attainable, given enough time and consistency of purpose. Let's look at an amazing example of perseverance.

In late 1996, American pro cyclist Lance Armstrong learned that he had testicular cancer. That the disease could attack someone so young and apparently healthy was unbelievable. In fact, the day the announcement was made in the press, many cyclists, knowing how fit the former world champ and Tour de France stage winner was, refused at first to accept the news. However, in the ensuing days they came to understand that it was, indeed, true. Then it was learned that the cancer had spread to his lungs and brain. At this point, many counted Armstrong out, but not Lance.

Armstrong took on the hardest challenge of his young life. His spirit remained strong as he persisted through multiple surgeries and chemotherapy. By late winter, his doctors announced that the cancer was in recession.

Armstrong could have accepted the inevitable. Instead, he sought the best medical advice available and declared that he would win this contest in the same way he had won numerous races—by remaining focused and persevering using whatever means necessary. Throughout the ordeal he rode his bike. Recreational riders with baby carriers passed him on the hills, he joked, but he remained steadfast in his desire to race again. As of this writing, he appears well on his way to returning to the peloton.

Don't give up on yourself. The question for your big cycling challenges isn't "Can I achieve them?" but rather "How long will it take?" Some goals may stretch you to your limits, and perhaps beyond, but those are the ones that produce the greatest pride.

R Is for Respect

Why is it we enjoy the company of some people, but not others? Although most of us have limited contact with pro athletes, you may find that some are more likable than others. Why is that? There's something different about the people we are attracted to. They don't have a big head, but that's not all. They have a healthy regard not only for their accomplishments, but also for ours. They make us feel good about ourselves.

Take American pro mountain biker Susan DeMattei, for example. In 1996, DeMattei won the bronze medal in the Atlanta Olympics. This was a truly historic occasion, given that it was the first time the mountain bike cross-country race was part of the Olympics. She had every right to feel pride in her accomplishment. Some might have become aloof and distant after such an achievement, but not DeMattei. She remained the same cheerful person who talked with everyone and showed a genuine interest in their accomplishments. Although they may not have an Olympic medal, other people's accomplishments are no less important to DeMattei.

For the successful cyclist, pride in personal achievements is necessary, but this comes easily for most. It's the accomplished rider who shows respect for others, including the competition, that we most admire. These people, by their actions say, "You're important, too."

It isn't always easy to show respect for others. After all, some are, well, different. Some are strong riders. Some aren't. They train differently. They eat different foods. They go to a different church, or no church. They have different values. They're younger or older, fatter or skinnier, taller or shorter. They're just different. The rider with healthy pride accepts the differences in others as necessary for making the sport, and even the world, better. How boring life would be if everyone was the same. Trying to make everyone just like you is sure to cause frustration and limit your circle of friends and supporters.

Respect is contagious. If you accept others for what they are and don't try to change them to fit your mold, they'll do the same for you. You will both accomplish more. There is no more powerful aid in achieving goals than the support of others. If you want success, you must first help others succeed.

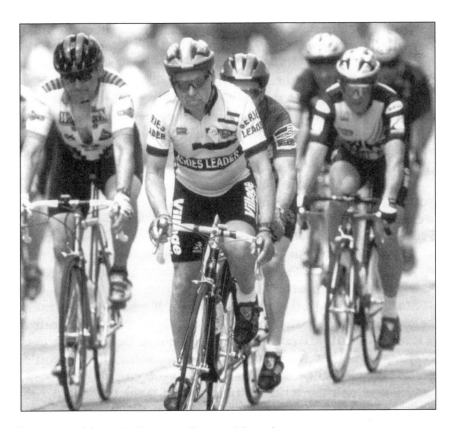

Races provide a challenge unlike anything else.

I Is for Intensity

If you've been riding for several years, it's easy to just go through the motions. Training and riding become a habit. In some ways, that's good as it means fitness is an integral part of your life. On the other hand, riding without purpose or regard for outcome is a sure way to start the downhill spiral we call getting old. A low level of emotional intensity for cycling, as with anything else in life, means boredom and an eventual loss of interest. Soon you're riding less and spending more time inactive. The less you ride, the less you want to ride.

If you truly love cycling, something must change to get you out of this spiral, to reestablish pride in your cycling accomplishments. Go back to your roots in the sport. Remember when you were first starting to ride a lot? Every day on the bike was enjoyable. Riding on the road or trail was like being a kid again. Getting more fit for riding was not a task or burden; it was a natural outgrowth of having fun. Then came new challenges such as tours, centuries, and perhaps races. With every new challenge came the motivation to ride stronger. The stronger you got, the more you wanted. If riding is no longer like that for you, it's time for a new challenge.

New challenges are scary. They mean possibly exposing your weaknesses to others and failing to succeed. When you were younger these weren't such a big deal. Why are they now? Probably because you've accepted a notion of who you are and what you do based on years of protecting self-esteem. It's time to let go of some of this defensiveness and take a risk, albeit safely and in measured doses at first.

Start by taking on a new challenge. If you've never raced before, that may be the challenge, or maybe it's a bike tour of a foreign country. Another challenge could be a double century, or even an Ironman-distance triathlon. Once you've picked the challenge, learn as much as you can about it. Read books and ask for written information from the event promoter, if there is one. Most importantly, talk to others who have done what you're thinking about doing. Pick their brains. Ride with them. The more you learn, the easier it is to see yourself achieving the goal.

Perhaps your lack of intensity, however, doesn't need a complete change of challenges. Maybe all you need is to rekindle your love affair with the bike within your area of interest. The key is still challenge and new horizons. This may mean new or even harder events than you've done before, or it could be as simple as riding with different people. Join a cycling club or ask about group rides at bike shops in the area. Get involved with others who are excited and intense about riding.

Whatever you do, decide it's time to quit going through the motions of riding. At the end of each day, ask if today was a waste or if you lived it with intensity. Did you feel challenged? Did you learn something new? Are you proud of today's accomplishments?

D Is for Daring

Cyclists who are proud of their accomplishments are also willing to take an occasional calculated gamble. Starting an event like a century or a race means dealing with risk, especially the risk that failure will result. The failure may range from not winning to not finishing. We're also afraid of the pain and discomfort that come with going far and fast. Standing tall to the little voice in your head warning you not to do it is what creates the greatest pleasure in achievement. Merely confronting the challenge head on, whether you ultimately succeed or not, is usually all that you need to bolster pride.

Overcoming fear isn't easy, and in fact, sports psychologists say that a little is good. A bit of anxiety steels you for the complaining, even screaming, muscles that will happen in every physical challenge like cycling.

Too much anxiety, however, is a problem. Excessive anxiety is the reason nearly everyone goes out too fast at the start of a race, century, or tour, then struggles to the finish line hours later. It's even possible to psych-up for a short event like a criterium or track race, then start so ambitiously that the pain of an injury goes away, only to reappear after the race with a vengeance and the loss of several days or weeks of training.

So, what can you do to get just the right amount of starting-line stress, but not too much? Here are some ways to keep the little voice in your head talking softly as you prepare for a new challenge.

Rehearse the course and conditions. There's nothing like having been there before to calm your nerves. In the weeks before an event, ride on the course, or parts of it, in training. If that's not possible, learn all you can about the course profile and find something that comes close. Train in similar, anticipated weather such as heat or wind when possible. Ride at the same time of day as the event. Prepare for the unique challenges of the event, such as uphill, downhill, wind, heat, cold, humidity, or early and late starts.

Rehearse the effort. Most past-50 cyclists spend too much time doing long, slow distance and not enough time practicing pace. Is it any wonder that the start of an event looks like a stampede of fourth graders heading for the playground at recess, with the finish resembling bedtime at the old folks home? How much time do you spend riding at your goal pace? If you're like most of us, not enough.

Rehearse mentally. While riding, sometimes rehearse in your head how you're going to concentrate on smooth pedaling technique in the event, how you'll pay close attention to your breathing and energy levels, and what adjustments you'll make if things aren't going well. Mental skills take at least as much practice as physical skills.

Develop a routine. The week of the big event, the night before, and the morning of it should become a habit—no thinking. The more nervous you get or the newer the challenge is for you, the more important this is. What will you eat and drink and when? When will you go to bed? What will you wear? When will you leave for the start site? Leave as little of this to chance as you possibly can. Practice will reduce much of the anxiety.

Have a preride ritual. The warm-up before an event should always be the same, no matter where you are or how important the event is. Practice the warm-up at least once a week to make it so routine that you can do it without thinking: automatic. A good time to do this is before your hardest training ride of the week.

Act as if. Whenever you feel the starting-line stress rising, act *as if* you were under control. That's what all the calm-looking riders are doing before an event. They're scared, too, only they don't show it. Move slowly, relax your belly, and act as if you were going for a workout with some friends.

Some of these tips may prove more helpful for meeting new cycling challenges than others. Use the ones you find most effective at reducing the fear, while allowing the mind to stay in tune with what's really important—riding the bike.

E Is for Enthusiasm

The rider who believes in his or her ability has a noticeable enthusiasm for cycling, but more important, for life in general. Enthusiasm results from enjoying the many tasks in life, cycling included. It's even a good barometer of what is going on with your riding and can tell you, or more likely, tell others if you're riding too much. Enjoyment is one of the first things to go when the balance between stress and rest is out of whack. It's easy to get so focused on riding, especially when preparing for an important event, that everything else, including family and friends, are relegated to lower priorities. Coaches can often tell when a rider is overreaching by simply hearing the enthusiasm level of the athlete's voice. At the extreme end, when overtraining, a cyclist will sound dull with no voice inflection or emotion.

The enthusiastic rider smiles, praises others, and avoids complaining and criticizing. When you adopt these behaviors, you tell others, "I'm so confident of who I am that I can unconditionally accept you." This attitude bolsters those around you, producing greater enthusiasm and better cycling performances for all.

Nothing says more about attitude than outward signs of happiness. The problem is, we don't always feel like smiling.

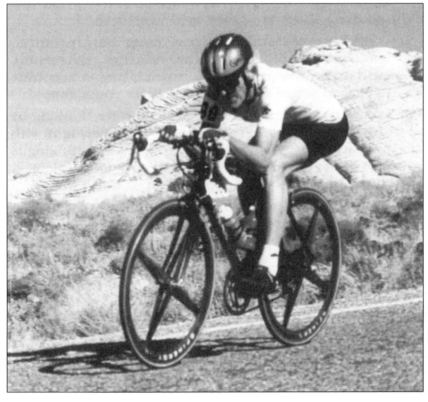

Snow Canyon, St. George, Utah, at the 1995 World Masters Huntsman's Games. Dick Finch finishes first among the 60-64 year olds.

The key, as described before, is to act as if. Act as if you're happy, and you'll soon be happy. Fake it till you make it.

The Confident Cyclist

If we could get inside the minds of cyclists who fully believe in their abilities, who have a no-limits outlook on life, we'd discover some unique attitudes. Their way of thinking helps produce consistently good rides under all conditions. Sports psychologist Gary Faris describes seven attitudes of such confident athletes.

1. Before and during an event, confident cyclists focus their thinking on what they want to happen, not what they are afraid might happen. They visualize success and talk positively about what they want to achieve.

2. Confident cyclists take charge of things that are controllable and let go of aspects of the event they can't control, such as weather conditions. Instead, they concentrate on how to adjust to the uncontrollable conditions.

3. Confident cyclists take charge of negative thinking by quickly noticing it, stopping it, then replacing it with positive thoughts. They know that positive thinking is not telling yourself a lie, but rather an optimistic look at the truth.

4. Obstacles are turned into opportunities by confident cyclists. They get excited by tough situations. When things don't go according to the plan, they reach deeper, to get more out of themselves. They try when others might fold.

5. Confident cyclists quickly and calmly let go of mistakes and refocus on the situation at hand. Mistakes are in the past. They're over and can't be changed. It's time to move on to the next challenge. They use mistakes as welcomed opportunities to learn something about the sport and improve themselves.

6. Confident cyclists know how to find fun and enjoyment in cycling, the kind of joy that comes with hard work, intensity, and challenge.

7. Confident cyclists take pride in themselves. This is not solely based on performance, but on all that goes into training, steady effort, and knowing who they are and why they ride.

Taking the lead from confident cyclists' attitudes and adopting them into your riding will help you get more out of your abilities while getting more enjoyment from the sport. Begin by paying attention to your thinking, especially when it runs counter to these confidence indicators. Try to reshape your attitudes and behaviors to match these, and your riding will improve along with your confidence.

11

The Cycling Community

So far this book has brought together several elements necessary for peak performance on a bike. Goals, training programs, recovery techniques, and mental skills all play important roles in successful cycling. However, you can go only so far with these tools. You also need something else—the support and assistance of others.

Riding a bike is by nature a solitary activity. Because of this, cycling attracts independent types who are willing to endure long hours in the saddle alone, with only a banana and two bits in a back pocket. In fact, the inability to ride alone probably indicates low motivation for the sport. Even for those who are happiest on their own, having the support and assistance of others is also important, perhaps even crucial for continued growth in the sport. Without a foundation built on the help of willing backers, you make little progress in any aspect of life, cycling included. Once you master the basics of physical and mental training, gathering around you a contingent of supporters who provide emotional encouragement, technical help, information, and motivation practically ensures success. Also, don't forget the fun factor. Without the pleasure of sharing your riding with others, cycling is likely to become drudgery.

Emotional Support

On the whole, cycling is a pleasure, but there are times when it becomes a drag, such as when you're bone weary from trying to do too much, your physical fitness isn't responding, or your riding just isn't up to par. It's during such times that the support of others is crucial. These are the tough times when those closest to you, your family and friends, can help. With their support, the passion for riding soon returns. If they're not on your side, the joy soon fades.

Family

Your spouse is your most important supporter. Without the enthusiastic encouragement of the person closest to you, the long hours of riding, recovering, tinkering on the bike, and traveling to and from events will take a toll. Every cyclist at some point, usually when worn out and with things not going well, wonders if it's all worth it and may even consider quitting. At times such as these, it's often spousal support that is the decisive factor.

The most supportive spouses are generally those who also participate in cycling. Empathy can come only from a spouse who has experienced firsthand what it's like to love the sport, yet go through tough times with it. Such a relationship is wonderfully effective for maintaining emotional support.

To help bolster such support, always look for ways to make cycling a family activity. Sharing training rides, trips to events, bicycling vacations, and enthusiasm for each other's accomplishments keeps the fun in cycling. Besides these direct links to the bike, support also comes from sharing housekeeping and meal preparation chores while your partner is riding or recovering.

Friends

There's no getting around it—cyclists are strange people. What else would a normal person call behaviors such as looking forward to several hours on a bicycle, avoiding sweet and tempting foods, and incessant talking about titanium components and seat-tube angles? Only other cyclists can fully understand such unusual conduct. Yet there are noncyclists who continue to associate with us and even feign interest in our discussions of personal cycling lore. They may not fully understand or even care about the important nuances of crank length, but they are always there when we need them. Such people are truly good friends whose support we must carefully nurture.

Support works both ways. You must be willing to go the extra mile for the friend who supports you. It may even occasionally mean the ultimate sacrifice—missing a workout. Being there for friends helps make life worth living. You receive in direct proportion to how much you give.

Technical Support

Preparing your body and your bike for peak performance is a complex endeavor. Bikes are becoming increasingly intricate, and breakthroughs in training and health sciences are happening at an exponential rate. It has become impossible for a rider to keep up with all that is known about maintaining and refining equipment, both mechanical and physiological. Specialists are the answer.

Bike Shops

Bike shops once were the unchallenged cultural center of the cycling universe. In the last 10 years, mail order has made profitability difficult in the bicycle retail industry, driving many marginal shops out of business. Those that are left have managed to carve a niche as a source of not only equipment, but also specialized services. The most valuable service for riders is the availability of a good bike mechanic. Someone who can expertly true a wheel, install a head set, overhaul a bottom bracket, and adjust a derailleur is hard to find. A bike shop can help you with bike setup to relieve unnecessary fatigue and even knee pain. This is also the place to go for event flyers and entry forms for tours, centuries, triathlons, duathlons, and mountain bike and road races. Often, the shop sponsors the event and can answer your questions about course terrain and other issues.

If you enjoy receiving these services, it behooves you to shop at your local bike store. You may find in most cases that prices are the same as those in the catalogs, especially when you consider the shipping costs. Even if you spend a couple dollars more, the services you receive are well worth the small extra expense.

Doctors

It wasn't too many years ago that when you saw a doctor about some cycling-related problem such as a sore knee, the only advice was to take two aspirin and stop riding a bicycle. Now, sports medicine is a booming business and destined to become even bigger as those of us in our 50s continue to push the envelope of physical fitness. A doctor who understands the intricacies of dealing with sports injury, and equally important, why you ride a bike, is a valuable asset. Just as a good mechanic keeps your bike in top shape, a good doctor can keep your body operational also.

The past-50 cyclist needs two types of doctors. First, find a family practitioner who rides a bike or at least is active in sports. Avoid those who smoke, are obese, or think that athletics is only for kids. Don't hesitate to interview the prospective physician just as you would any other employee. It will cost a few dollars to meet with him or her before committing, but the expense is worth it in the long run.

The second type of doctor you may need is a sports medicine specialist. There are fewer options in this case, but people in this field of medicine are generally sports buffs themselves and won't try to talk you out of continuing to cycle. Instead, they will look for ways to treat and rehabilitate injuries that your family doctor isn't equipped to handle.

You may even have a reason for a third type of doctor—a podiatrist. Many physical problems cyclists, and especially triathletes and duathletes, experience from the knee down are from poor foot mechanics. Suspect this whenever pain, especially knee or ankle pain, refuses to go away despite a concerted effort to refine bike setup and treat the symptoms. Often a podiatrist can examine your feet clipped into the pedals or unshod and see a problem you can easily correct with a shoe insert.

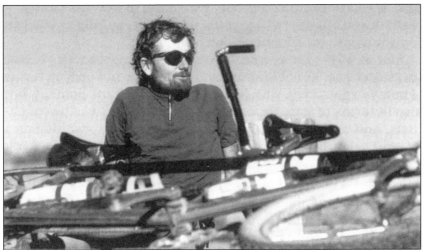

© 1995 Richard Etchberger

Cool, calm and relaxed: A rider enjoys a rest off his bike.

The best sources when looking for a specific type of doctor or experiencing an injury are other riders. Ask around. You may be surprised at how common your ache or pain is. Someone else has probably had the same complaint and found effective medical help. Riders also keep up on who are the most understanding family doctors in your area.

Coaches

Most amateur riders aren't aware that there are coaches available who can evaluate abilities and design a program that will produce peak fitness at just the right times. Many of those who do know of cycling coaches assume they work only with young, elite, and professional riders. It's not true.

The field of coaching is growing larger every year. What was once a part-time hobby for some has become a full-time profession for many. The USA Cycling Federation has encouraged this growth in the last few years by establishing a five-tiered program of certification for coaches in road, track, and mountain bike. The USA Triathlon Federation is working on a similar program. For information on finding a coach, contact the USA Cycling National Coaching Director (719-578-4581).

If you're new to the sport, it's best that your coach live near you so he or she can observe you riding and offer hands-on tips. If you're beyond the first two years of serious riding, it really doesn't matter where your coach lives, so long as you can communicate by telephone, fax, or E-mail.

Just as with your doctor, talk to two or three coaches before you select one. You'll find many differences, not only in terms of how you get along, which is the most important element, but also in terms of fees, experience, advanced degrees, certifications, and procedures. A good coach loves the sport, listens a lot and talks little, sees the positive side of even the worst situations, and is obviously concerned with your progress as a cyclist. He or she should consider your riding history, goals, and lifestyle when designing a program. Stay away from coaches who hand out the same workouts to everyone. No two people should train exactly the same way.

Besides designing and refining a training program, some coaches also provide advice on equipment purchases, diet, event strategy, mental skills development, and even motivational support. In fact, just having a coach is usually great for motivation.

Informational Support

The late 20th century saw an explosion of knowledge such as the world has never known. The same goes for information on cycling equipment, training, and nutrition. What you discovered last year is now old hat, and what you learned five years ago is ancient. Staying worldly wise, even in cycling, requires having good sources of information. It's not possible to stay in touch with all of them, so pick a couple from the following to keep up with change.

Cyberspace Cycling

The Internet is undoubtedly the fastest growing segment of the information market. Newsgroups, bulletin boards, Web sites, chat rooms, online magazines, and live talks by experts abound. It's almost mind-boggling. There are thousands of locations from around the world on topics as diverse as the Bicycling Hall of Fame, helmet safety, and tours of China's Hunan Province.

A great deal of information is available on the Internet related to aging and performance. One of the best is a Norwegian Web site called Masters Athletes Physiology and Performance (MAPP). MAPP is the brainchild of Stephen Seiler, PhD, an American exercise physiologist teaching at Agder College in Kristiansand, Norway. His passions are rowing, cycling, cross-country skiing, and improving the performance of aging athletes. His Web site is full of understandable information on physiology, training, nutrition, and equipment. In addition, he has links to other good informational sites. You can access this Web site at **http://www.krs.hia.no/ ~stephens/index.html.**

Another way to keep up with what's going on in your corner of the cycling world is with mailing lists through the VeloNet, an electronic information desk for cyclists. Mailing lists are

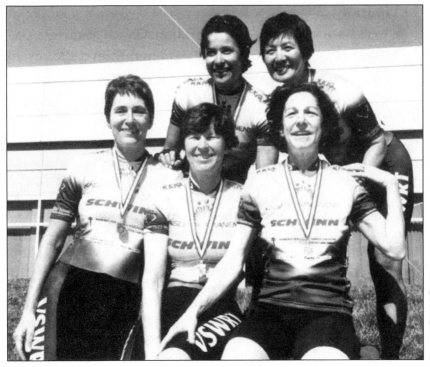

© 1997 David Powers

California criterium medal winners from the Valley Spokesmen Women's Race Team.

E-mail announcements, discussions, advice, opinions, and experiences of cyclists on a wide range of well-defined cycling topics. To get a complete list of mailing lists available on cycling, send an E-mail to **majordomo@cycling.org** with the single word "Lists" in the message body. Besides the list, you will receive instructions about how to sign on to and off of a list of your choice.

A few sample lists currently available on VeloNet mailing lists are the following:

- Coaching—coaching discussions for racers
- Marketplace—discussions on buying bicycles and components
- Masters—discussions about masters racing for USCF and NORBA events
- Mtb—general discussions about mountain biking
- Touring—general discussion on all aspects of bicycle touring
- Trifed-smw—Triathlon Federation, South Midwest, USA
- Ultra—discussions regarding ultramarathon cycling events
- Uscf-results—race results for USCF events

Magazines

The availability of magazines and media coverage on any topic reflect the interests of society. When bicycling is popular, the cycling press flourishes. This was evident at the end of the last century when bicycles were rapidly becoming the major mode of transportation. During this golden age of bicycling, media coverage of the bike was unparalleled, with entire sections of newspapers devoted to them, much as is done for automobiles today. In the last 25 years there has been a reemergence of cycling popularity, and the magazine industry shows it. Between 1972 and 1994, more than 20 bicycle periodicals started. In the late 1980s and early 1990s, the Audit Bureau of Circulations reported that cycling magazines had the greatest growth of subscribers in all categories. Two of the top four in this fast-growth category were *Mountain Bike Action* and *VeloNews*.

Today there are magazines available on touring, ultradistance riding, technology, fitness, road and mountain bike racing, off-road riding, recumbents, tandems, triathlon, and bike equipment. If there's a subject related to cycling that suits your fancy, there's probably a magazine that covers it. One of the biggest, and the best for general interest in cycling, is *Bicycling*, a glossy published by Rodale Press of Emmaus, Pennsylvania. Monthly issues include a broad range of topics such as training, touring, equipment purchases, racing, industry news, repair and maintenance, medical issues, commuting, and general interest. Past feature stories have included aging and performance.

Other popular magazines with more narrow focuses are *Bicycle Guide, Fitness Cycling, Inside Triathlon, Mountain Bike, Road Bike Action, Triathlete*, and *Winning*. Subscribing to one or more of these publications will keep you in touch with the latest developments in the sport.

Due to their quick production time and propensity for keeping an ear the ground, newsletters are a good choice for the past-50 cyclist who wants to keep up with a particular area of interest. Several are available. A good general-interest newsletter for those who cross train is *MastersSports*, a monthly publication devoted to aging athletes. Its eight pages pack in a lot of current information about fitness, training, competition, and sports medicine. To subscribe call 800-562-1973.

One of the best newsletters for the racer is *Performance Conditioning for Cycling (PCF)*. Its editorial board includes such cycling luminaries as sports scientist Edmund Burke, national team coach Chris Carmichael, strength specialist Vern Gambetta, cycling biomechanics expert Andy Pruitt, and others. *PCF* includes leading edge training concepts of the country's top coaches written with the athlete in mind. It's a full-color, glossy, eight-page publication that's printed nine times a year. For subscription information, call 800-578-4636.

The Silver Streak is a newsletter out of San Diego written for the past-50 woman cyclist. It includes editorials, results, encouragement, and cycling tips from experienced riders and experts such as *Bicycling* magazine Advisory Board members

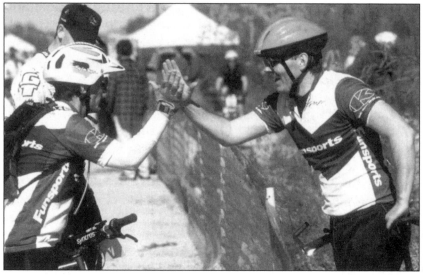

Lasting competition and friendships: A high-five to the cycling community.

© 1996 Richard Etchberger

Camilla Buchanan, MD, and Arnie Baker, MD. Call 619-583-6647 to subscribe.

There are a host of nonprofit organizations devoted to narrow aspects of cycling that each put out a newsletter. By joining one of these in your area of interest, you'll not only keep abreast of what's going on in the field, but also directly support cycling. See Cycling Organizations for a partial listing of resource groups.

CYCLING ORGANIZATIONS

The following nonprofit groups each support a specific facet of the sport of cycling and provide members with information and resources. The list is far from complete, but includes many leading organizations.

Adventure Cycling Association

P.O. Box 8308

Missoula, MT 59807

406-721-1776

Formerly known as Bikecentennial, ACA offers routes for self-contained tours within the United States and provides supported and guided tours covering about 45 miles per day. Some of their tours are coast to coast.

Bicycle Federation of America
1506 21st St. NW, Ste. 200
Washington, DC 20036
202-463-6622
The Federation promotes bikes for transportation and lobbies Congress for greater support. It provides information and statistics on bike use.

International Human-Powered Vehicle Association
P.O. Box 51255
Indianapolis, IN 46251
317-876-9478
The IHPVA organizes an annual competition for human-powered vehicles of all types and promotes innovation in human-powered conveyance.

International Mountain Bike Association
P.O. Box 7578
Boulder, CO 80306-7578
303-545-9011
IMBA promotes environmentally responsible and socially conscious off-road riding.

League of American Bicyclists
190 West Ostend St., Ste 120
Baltimore, MD 21230
410-539-3399
Founded in 1880 as the League of American Wheelmen, this is the oldest bicycling organization in the country. The League promotes cycling as transportation and serves commuting, touring, and recreational cyclists.

National Off-Road Bicycling Association
1750 East Boulder
Colorado Springs, CO 80909
719-578-4717
NORBA is an extension of USA Cycling and the national governing body of off-road racing.

United States Cycling Federation
1 Olympic Plaza
Colorado Springs, CO 80909
719-578-4581
USCF is an extension of USA Cycling and the national governing body of road and track racing.

USA Cycling
1 Olympic Plaza
Colorado Springs, CO 80909
719-578-4581
This organization is charged by Congress with the responsibility of overseeing bicycle racing in the United States.

USA Triathlon
P.O. Box 15820
Colorado Springs, CO 80935
719-597-9090
USAT is the governing body for triathlon and duathlon in the United States.

Women's Cycling Coalition
P.O. Box 7313
Loveland, CO 80537
970-669-5940
The WCC promotes racing and recreational riding for women.

Motivational Support

There's one thing sure about cyclists—they enjoy the company of other cyclists, especially when it's time for a long ride. That's because cycling is a unique sport in the world of endurance athletics. Few long-distance sports demand such long workouts as are routine in cycling. Workouts that last three to five hours are not uncommon for the rider training for a century, tour, or race. A steady diet of such rides done solo causes mind-numbing boredom. A training partner or, better yet, a group is the best therapy.

Clubs

Due largely to this need for riding companions, cycling has always had a strong, local-club system in this country. A call to a local bike shop will help you locate a club devoted to recreation or racing, and to road or mountain biking. These clubs generally have regularly scheduled weekend rides. Larger clubs divide these rides into ability groups with different planned distances and speeds. In the summer months, some offer twilight criterium races. Most hold monthly meetings with speakers and provide a newsletter with helpful tips.

There are even clubs for past-50 cyclists. A good example is the Colorado Bicycle Racing Association for Seniors (CO-BRAS). The Denver chapter meets monthly and provides training rides, educational programs, and social events. Besides fellowship, the COBRAS also offer a six-week series of Wednesday-evening time trials in the Denver area that are open to the public and USCF racers. The club reaches well beyond the Colorado state lines, with members from California to Massachusetts. For more information on the COBRAS call 303-320-4413.

Training Partners

If there isn't a club in your area, finding other cyclists of similar ability for a weekly ride will do wonders for your enthusiasm when it comes time to head out for several hours. Again, a local bike shop frequented by riders with interests similar to yours is the place to begin looking. Many shops provide bulletin boards on which you can place a looking-for-training-partners note.

If you're a racer, besides long rides, it can also be helpful to do interval and sprint workouts with a companion of similar ability. This will provide the motivation you need to push the envelope in these tough workouts. For a mountain biker, training with a more experienced rider is a good way to quickly refine technical handling skills, a crucial aspect of off-road riding. Seeing how an accomplished rider lifts the front wheel, takes a line on tricky terrain, or climbs on loose soil will accelerate your learning curve.

In the winter months, indoor trainer workouts with a training partner help the time go faster and boost the quality of such rides. You can design your own indoor workouts or purchase video tapes from Cycle Ops (800-261-8405) that will provide structure and motivation. In addition, spin classes are offered by many health clubs. These are typically led by experienced riders and provide motivational support. The bikes they use are far superior to the old stationary bikes you may be familiar with and give a real-world feel to such workouts.

12

Fit Forever

Cycling is one of the most common of all human activities. It's been estimated that only 10 percent of the world's residents can afford a car, but for a full 80 percent a bike is within their means. One authority estimates that there are about one billion bikes on the planet, one for every six people, with most used for transportation (70 percent), some for recreation (29 percent), and a few for competition (1 percent). In the United States, where the automobile is king, the transportation and recreation percentages common throughout most of the world are reversed, with about 70 percent of American cyclists riding primarily for recreation.

Regardless of age, gender, ability, experience, or even equipment, people commute, commune, and compete on bicycles. The Bicycle Institute of America estimates that there are approximately 100-million cyclists in this country with most being women (55 percent) and adults (55 percent). But motivation must be a problem for many, as the Institute has determined that only about a third of these users actually get on their bikes at least once a week. That's too bad, as the bike has the potential to solve many of our nation's problems, including traffic congestion; air and noise pollution; deteriorating roadways; productive use of land; obesity; and premature death from causes such as automobile accidents, heart disease, and some cancers. If more of us regularly got our bikes out of the garage and used them to run errands, race, or just ride for improved fitness and fun, this would be a better country.

But this is preaching to the choir—you already use a bike in one of these ways or you wouldn't be reading this book. That's not to say that your motivation for riding never varies. Even for the most serious riders, there are times when getting on the bike is an unattractive option. This may happen more regularly than you'd like. Perhaps it's time to try something different, to use your bike in a new way by crossing into another discipline of cycling. Are you a racer but have never toured by bicycle, or a commuter who has never raced? It may be time to consider one or more alternatives for how you usually ride.

Staying Motivated

Physical challenges such as long rides and big hills aside, there are some days when getting on the bike is more of a mental challenge. At such times the company of friends is a sure cure. Knowing there are others waiting to ride with you is great motivation for most. Another strategy is to make cycling such an integral part of your daily life that thinking about it is never an issue. For many, commuting by bike is the way to accomplish that. Others find that the carrot-on-the-stick method is their best motivator, especially a competitive carrot. Competition is enticing and frightening at the same time, an interesting mixture that fuels the desire to ride.

It may be time for adding variety to your cycling by adopting a new use for your bike that may ignite the flame of enthusiasm for riding. This doesn't necessarily mean giving up what's become a long-standing relationship between you and your bike. It may only take a little variety from time to time to spark the fire.

Commuting

American visitors arriving by train in the Italian city of Ferrara, a Medieval city on the Po River in the country's northeast plain, are quick to notice the sea of bicycles outside the bustling train station. Thousands of bikes are racked waiting for their owners to return at the end of the day from work in nearby cities. In this ancient, walled city, the bicycle is the king of the road. The people of Ferrara travel everywhere by bike. The morning rush-hour commute is pedal-to-pedal traffic, with women in dresses and high heels and men wearing business suits and ties. People talk on cellular telephones or drink coffee as they roll along. Mothers with two children aboard take the youngsters to day care and to school. Grandmothers on bikes loaded with groceries after a morning trip to the baker, butcher, and fruit shop negotiate Ferrara's bustling streets. When it rains, the bicycles sprout umbrellas, and the two-wheeled commute continues. When it's chilly, heavy coats are everywhere. Nothing perturbs these people or keeps them from their daily rounds—all done on basic, but sturdy bicycles.

Ferrara is designed with the bicycle in mind. The busy main street has separated, one-way lanes for bikes that are kept in the same excellent condition as the automobile-dedicated streets. Parking racks are evident at all the major destinations, and cars are forbidden in the central shopping area. At the rail station, a visitor can rent a bike for the day to see the city's many historic sites or to conduct business.

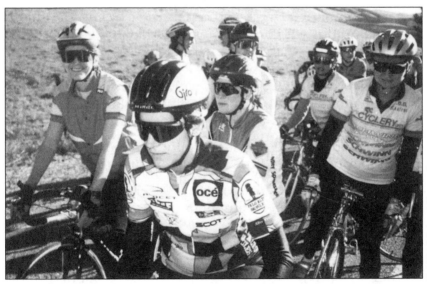

© 1994 Michael Alexander

At her first race, Dianna Waggoner (far left) flashes a nervous grin.

There is definitely a love affair with the bike, and the benefits are obvious. The citizens' penchant for traveling on two wheels is evident in their level of fitness, regardless of age. Obesity is so rare in Ferrara that overweight people are easily confirmed as tourists. The air is also clean, another benefit of a city that travels largely by bike. The only traffic congestion in Ferrara is in the bike lanes, where commuters are counted in the hundreds per city block, instead of in the dozens as in car-addicted American cities of the same size.

Although Ferrara is an eye-opening exception, Europe, the birthplace of the bicycle, is generally more bike-friendly and commuter-conscious than the United States. Old European cities such as Ferrara grew with walking in mind, and most people still live close to markets and workplaces. In the United States, many cities developed based on travel by car, especially in the West where you find the youngest cities. Housing and the usual destinations, such as shopping centers and office buildings, are widely separated and connected by roadways designed, often exclusively, for high-speed auto use. A gallon of gasoline, an expensive commodity in Europe, costs less in the United States than a gallon of bottled water. America has a love affair with the automobile that borders on addiction.

If you commute to work and run errands by car, the shift to bike commuting will change your perceptions. The car isolates the driver from other people and sanitizes the process of transportation. Travel by bike encourages interaction, not only with other people, but also with the environment.

Bike commuting isn't all a bed of roses, however. For one thing, most U.S. cities woefully lack designated roadways for bikes. It seems that bike pathways are a chicken-and-egg situation: Planners don't see the need for better cycling roadways, although they are cheaper to build and maintain than auto roadways, because few Americans commute by bike. However, cycling is unpopular, in part at least, because of poor bike facilities.

Commuting by bike requires the rider to become accomplished at dealing with obstacles such as narrow roadway shoulders, loose gravel, parked cars, potholes, slotted sewer grates, and debris. All this detracts from the cycling experience and makes commuting difficult and even unsafe.

Weather also presents problems. It's interesting, however, that what is tolerable weather for commuting varies from region to region. In California, for example, cyclists seldom ride when the forecast calls for rain, but those in Oregon continue to commute anyway, making adjustments in their clothing and equipment. In Colorado snow doesn't deter the avid cyclist, but in Arizona temperatures below 60 degrees are considered too cold.

Overcoming such obstacles makes bike commuting a great challenge, depending on the conditions in your area, but a challenge worth overcoming. Whether you're into bike touring, fitness, or racing, the benefits of getting around on a bike are many. Riding to and from work and errands is an excellent way to get in good aerobic shape. The primary advantage of bike commuting is efficient use of time. Because you have to go to certain daily destinations regardless of mode, travel by bike allows you to gain something valuable from the trip. Additionally, once there, you don't have to search for a parking space or pay to park. During rush hour, it's faster going across town on a bike than in a car, and it's far cheaper to travel by bike. All told, there are more advantages to commuting by bike than there are disadvantages. In fact, many elite racers, such as Ken Bostick, a member of the U.S. cycling team at the 1996 Atlanta Olympics, commute by bike regularly. You can do it, too.

Your enjoyment and the benefits you gain from bike commuting depend greatly on the equipment you use. A mountain bike or *cross* bike (a hybrid design incorporating many of the best features of road and mountain bikes) may be the best option, because they provide greater comfort and stability with their upright position and wider tires. Installing smooth tires designed for road use will make the travel easier than knobbies, but if you live in the snow belt, a second set of knobby wheels will improve riding on snow. You'll also want fenders installed to keep wet roads from messing up clothing. Adding battery-powered lights both front and rear will provide safety should you occasionally bike when it's dark. These work better than wheel-generator types, which glow at low intensity when riding slowly. To carry briefcases or purchases add panniers, wire baskets, or a rear rack. It's also wise to purchase a heavy-duty lock.

Commuting to work by bike requires judicious planning, especially if the trip takes more than 20 minutes. For the short commutes you can ride slowly on the way to work so you don't break a sweat. This is a relaxing yet invigorating way to start the day and doesn't generally require a change of clothes once you arrive. After work you can change into workout clothing and get a hard, fitness ride back home. For the longer rides, it's best if you have a place to shower and change clothes at your workplace or nearby.

Getting in the extra miles by commuting will build greater aerobic fitness without taking any more time out of your day. It's a great way to augment your fitness while carrying out the necessary but mundane task of traveling around town. Most find that once they start doing it, the obstacles are easily overcome and they're more alert and productive at work.

Camaraderie

Sharing a ride with friends makes cycling more enjoyable. Perhaps that's why there are so many bike clubs and group rides. Some rides are organized by clubs or individuals and generally have structure, such as division into smaller subgroups by ability or age. Other rides just happen and are unstructured gatherings that involve racing. In some cases, these latter rides have been going on so long that no one remembers how or why they started. Such is the case with the Oval ride in Fort Collins, Colorado.

Every Sunday at 11 A.M., cyclists gather at Oval Drive on the Colorado State University campus and head out on a route that has been used for years. In the spring more than a hundred riders may show up. This ride, and many around the country like it, is not popular with the residents along the course or with the police, as it takes over the roads and charges ahead through stop lights and stop signs. For years there has been an ongoing confrontation between the police and this group. It's best to avoid such rides.

Organized rides are preferred, especially those sponsored by a club. Some clubs require membership to join the fun, but most don't. Nonmembers may be asked to sign a waiver or pay a small fee, however. These rides are a great way to meet others with a similar interest and get in a workout at the same time.

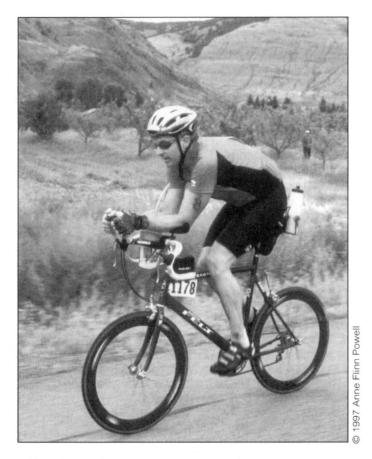

© 1997 Anne Flinn Powell

Live long. Train hard. Enjoy!

However, be sure to find out what the purpose of the ride is before showing up. Some are intended strictly as endurance builders, with someone in charge of keeping the speed at a predetermined level. Others are mainly for social interaction and may include stops along the way, or at the end, for breakfast or pizza. Many head for the hills and others keep it flat. Some may include intervals or racing. Ask what to expect before showing up.

Charities often sponsor group rides to raise funds. These include distances as short as 15 miles or tours that last several days. Such events may have a dozen participants or several thousand. By joining you help a worthy cause while enjoying a supported ride.

CYCLING CALENDAR

Tired of doing the same old things? Looking for a getaway with your spouse and bike? Want to meet other cyclists and get the high-motivation juices flowing again? Here is a sampling of century rides, city tours, state tours, and mountain bike events that may inspire you.

Century Rides

Assault on Mount Mitchell. This North Carolina event held every year in the early summer features a 102-mile ride to the peak of the highest point east of the Rocky Mountains. It attracts some 1,500 riders intent on making it up the 5,000 vertical feet to the top. For information contact the Spartanburg Freewheelers, Box 6161, Spartanburg, South Carolina 29304.

Davis Double Century. If 100 miles just isn't long enough for you, how about trying 200? This northern California event is held in late May. The animals will do it in less than 10 hours. For information contact the Davis Bicycle Club, 610 3rd Street, Davis, California 95616.

Leadville Trail 100. There aren't too many off-road centuries around. This one, on the single-track fire roads and dirt roads, is more of a race. There's a 12-hour finish cutoff. It's held in mid-August in Leadville, Colorado, with the trails peaking higher than 10,000 feet in places. There's an entry limit and it fills up fast every year. For information call 719-486-3502.

City Tours

El Tour de Tucson. Four main routes of 111, 75, 50, or 25 miles encircle the city of Tucson for this November, one-day event. *Bicycling* magazine has named it one of the top-10 centuries and the city of Tucson as one of best for cycling in the country. Putting those two together makes a good ride. Expect about 6,000 riders of all ages and abilities. For information contact PBAA, Inc., 630 N. Craycroft, Suite 141, Tucson, Arizona 85711.

The Great Five Boro Bike Tour. Starting and ending on Staten Island, the tour weaves through Manhattan, Bronx, and Brooklyn on its 42-mile journey. More than 28,000 riders are expected for the early May ride each year. For information call 212-932-2453.

Tour de L'Ile de Montreal. This early June, 44-mile tour of the city of Montreal, Quebec, is considered the biggest gathering of cyclists in the world, according to the Guinness Book of Records. Expect about 45,000 riders of all abilities. For information call 514-521-8356.

State Tours

Biking Across Kansas. If you're looking for a flat tour, this is the one. However, just as Dorothy found in the Wizard of Oz, wind can be a problem in Kansas, so come prepared with aero bars. This is one of the oldest state tours in the country, dating back to 1975, and attracts about 1,000 riders for a week-long ride in early June. For information call 316-684-8184.

RAGBRAI (Register's Annual Great Bicycle Ride Across Iowa). Think Iowa is a boring place? See what happens there when you put a few thousand riders on the road for a week of touring, covering 500 miles in hot, hot July. This is one of the oldest and most popular across-state rides in the Union, and the entries are limited, so you'll have to sign up several months in advance. For information contact RAGBRAI, Box 622, Des Moines, Iowa 50303.

Ride the Rockies. Known as one of the toughest week-long state tours in the country, this 500-or-so-mile ride changes its course annually, but always includes lots of climbing in Colorado's Rocky Mountains. Held in July, it's big (about 2,000 riders) and selects riders by lottery. For information contact the Denver Post, Ride the Rockies, 1560 Broadway, Denver, Colorado 80202.

Mountain Bike

Canyonlands Fat Tire Festival. This mid-October, five-day celebration of mountain biking takes place in one the most scenic havens of trail riding—Moab, Utah. On the preceding weekend, the 24 Hours of Moab, a team relay event, attracts a strong field of racers. There are plenty of slickrock trails to ride every day near this high-desert city. For information call 801-375-3231.

Fat Tire Week. This isn't a ride, but a week in July of mountain bike-related fun and partying in Crested Butte, Colorado. This week of merriment pivots around a mountain bike race, group rides, and a relaxed attitude. For information contact Fat Tire Bike Week, Box 782, Crested Butte, Colorado 81224.

West Virginia Fat Tire Festival. Judging by this and the Crested Butte Fat Tire Week, you'd think that mountain bikers were a fun-loving group. You'd be right. In August the East Coast, fat-tire crowd comes together for racing, mountain bike clinics, music, and fun. For information contact Elk River Touring Center, Highway 219, Slatyfork, West Virginia 26291.

The biggest group ride in the world is the Tour de L'Ile in Montreal, which attracts upward of 40,000 cyclists for a 45-mile loop. Probably the oldest group ride is the Journée Velocio held each July near Saint-Etienne in France. Founded in 1922, the Journée attracts riders of all ages and abilities for a trip to the summit of the Col du Grand Bois, where a picnic is provided and the oldest riders are celebrated. As for fund-raisers, one of the most successful is the TransAmerica Bicycle Trek, sponsored by the American Lung Association. It raises about $1.5 million from its annual 3,357-mile tour from Seattle to Atlantic City, New Jersey.

To boost sagging motivation, find a group that matches your interests to ride with weekly or organize your own. This will provide the impetus to get you out the door, while making what is probably your longest ride of the week pass quickly. Consider targeting one or two noncompetitive group tours each year to give your cycling a focal point. Knowing that you have a certain number of weeks to get ready provides sure motivation.

Competition

If you find your motivation to ride waning from time to time, another effective way to rekindle the fire is to train for a race. Racers are among the most dedicated of cyclists, in part because competition is so intimidating and yet personally rewarding. Whether you win or finish well back in the field, you can't beat the thrill of accomplishment that comes from meeting the challenge of a race. It's sure to get your juices flowing again.

BRIEF HISTORY OF BIKE RACING

People have raced bicycles since the 1860s when a Parisian blacksmith first fitted cranks and pedals on a *swift walker*. The swift walker, developed by the German Karl von Drais in 1816, was a device that roughly resembled a bike on which the user sat and walked. As people have done with every mode of transportation ever developed, Europeans on swift walkers probably tested their speed against one another from time to time, but there are no records of competitions.

The first organized bike race was held in Paris on May 31, 1868. It was a 1,200-meter sprint won by Englishman James Moore in 3 minutes, 50 seconds. Later that year, the first race for women was conducted, also in Paris. The details were not recorded.

The following year, the first endurance bike competition pitted 109 riders, including 12 women, in a 76-mile race from Paris to

Rouen. James Moore also won this contest in 10 hours, 45 minutes, with an average speed of 7 miles per hour. An English lady, who remains unknown to this day, came in 22nd overall, topping the women's field in 17 hours.

In the 1870s, velocipede racing clubs formed in France and quickly spread to Italy and England, attracting spectators to a wide array of events. Popular races included the mile; the hour; the 24-hour; and cross-country, multiday competitions. About this time, cycling was also becoming popular in the United States as evidenced by the formation of the League of American Wheelmen (now the League of American Bicyclists) in 1880, which added a Racing Board the following year. By the 1890s, six-day races on the track were attracting upwards of 18,000 spectators to New York's Madison Square Garden. Before the turn of the century there were more than a thousand professional racers, including women, in America.

The Tour de France was born in 1903 as a six-stage race around France, covering 1,500 miles in 19 days. Of the 60 starters that first year, only a third made it back to Paris.

Bicycle racing continues to evolve. The most notable additions to the sport came out of California in the 1970s. In Marin County, in the hills near San Francisco, young men began to race their clunkers down the trails. The heavy-framed, fat-tired bikes that developed from this were a cross between BMX bikes and off-road motorcycles. In 1983 mountain biking, as it came to be known, became an organized sport with the establishment of the National Off-Road Bicycle Association (NORBA). There were 112 members that year. By the mid-1990s, NORBA boasted some 35,000 members and was a full Olympic event in the 1996 Atlanta Games.

About the same time that the mountain bike was invented, a handful of endurance athletes in southern California began combining cycling with running or swimming and the triathlon was born. In 1978 the first Ironman race was held in Hawaii. The 2000 Olympics in Sydney, Australia will include triathlon.

There are many types of bike races. On the road there are time trials, road races, criteriums, ultraendurance races, and even across-the-continent events. Off-road racing includes mountain bike cross-country and downhill, plus cyclocross. Triathlon and duathlon include bike portions that vary from 12 to 112 miles. Multisport races are also done off-road on mountain bikes. On the track there are many events to choose from, including the sprint, kilometer, and pursuit.

Of the many race possibilities, the most basic and the easiest to get started in is the time trial. This is an individual race against the clock in which riders start at 30-second or 1-minute intervals, and drafting is not allowed. The outcome is determined strictly by individual effort and not team strategy.

Besides the individual time-trial competitions conducted around the country by United States Cycling Federation (USCF) sanctioned clubs, this type of event is also at the core of mountain bike cross-country, triathlon, and duathlon racing. A fun way to get started in racing is to enter the team competition of a triathlon or duathlon with a friend or two.

Success in your first time-trial event, whether it's USCF, mountain bike, triathlon, or duathlon, depends largely on developing the most basic elements of cycling fitness—aerobic

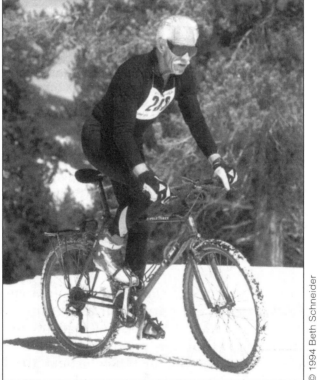

© 1994 Beth Schneider

The Snowman Triathlon in Copper Mountain, Colorado, challenges even the oldest of youngsters!

endurance, strength, and muscular endurance. Also important is a good sense of pacing.

Assuming that for the few weeks before starting this program you've been riding regularly and including hills, there are two areas to work on in the last 6 to 10 weeks before your first time trial. The first is a weekly muscular-endurance workout, including either cruise intervals or threshold rides. Both workouts are described in detail in chapter 4.

Pacing is a little different. Instead of training your body to go faster, you train your brain to hold back just the right amount. It's common in time trialing, especially the first one, for the rider to go out far too quickly, then struggle to finish the race. There's only one way to improve pacing and that's to practice it. Once every two weeks in the last two months before the race, set your bike up just as it will be for the race (this usually includes adding aero bars); then conduct your own six- to eight-mile time trial. Use a road that is mostly flat, has no stop streets, and light traffic. By improving your time on this course, you will soon develop a keen sense of pacing.

Use caution: When time trialing always keep your head up so you can see what's in front of you. Many riders have suffered severe head and spinal injuries by riding into the back of stopped cars with their heads down.

The day of the race, warm up for about 20 minutes with steadily increasing effort. Then do three or four 30- to 60-second accelerations up to race pace, with long, easy recovery spinning between them. When it's your turn to start, remember the pacing you've practiced and hold back a little. If you've rested in the last week to 10 days before as you should have, it will feel easy, and the temptation to go faster than practiced will be high. Ignore it. Stick with your plan. You'll be glad you did in the last few miles.

Down the Road

Staying fit forever may mean making changes in your cycling to match the changes taking place in your life. For example, you may have more free time now or even face early retirement. This newfound freedom provides the time to add another dimension to cycling in your life. Perhaps you're ready to take on a new challenge or do something you've dreamed of doing for years. In case you don't have a dream but are looking for a new adventure, a few are presented here. The possibilities are nearly endless; with a little imagination you can find just the adventure for you.

Create your own ageless goals:

- Ride across the country.
- Complete an Ironman or double century.
- Set a new personal best time for a century or a time trial.
- Improve your cycling by working with a coach or trainer.
- Write and self-publish a book on your cycling experiences and insights.
- Complete a bike tour of a foreign country.
- Ride in all 50 states.
- Complete 50 tours, centuries, or races.

Another way to stay active and ageless is to give something back to the sport:

- Volunteer to work at least one event a year.
- Start a bike club in your area.
- Set up a cycling Web site on the Internet.
- Be a big brother or sister to a novice cyclist.
- Teach bicycle safety to kids.
- Take a leadership position in your club.
- Organize and direct an event.

Or how about combining your career experience and interest in cycling into a new vocation:

- Sales, mechanic—work in a bike shop.
- Manager—manage a bike shop.
- Business owner, investment manager—buy a bike shop.
- Travel agent—organize and lead bike tours.
- Lawyer—become an agent for professional cyclists.
- Physician, physiologist—coach or train cyclists.
- Marketing, public relations—work for or start a cycling camp.

Getting Older—Getting Better

Throughout this book there is a strong emphasis on remaining youthful. This does not imply a superficial or cosmetic *appearance* of youth. It is instead an emphasis on maintaining a youthful outlook on life, one that seeks the future rather than dwelling on the past. The youthful cyclist past the age of 50 doesn't think with age-limiting attitudes, but considers the many possibilities and new opportunities that are presented daily. The youthful past-50 cyclist is in tune with the art of enjoying life and wringing the most from every day.

The art of having fun in cycling is continually seeking and conquering new challenges—neither too easy nor out of reach. This is the hunger of human motivation. We're each turned on by these delicious uncertainties, these new challenges that we have the potential to master.

We don't race or push the limits of a century or tour to conquer the course or defeat other riders, but rather for the experience. The calculated risk that comes from riding near your perceived limits of endurance and speed allow you to emerge from the event euphoric and somehow better for having experienced it. The quest of cycling is self-fulfillment, not victory. Each new, challenging event offers this opportunity for self-discovery and satisfaction.

When we no longer seek new challenges that explore our limits, when riding becomes a mundane routine, we grow old. George Burns perhaps said it best: "You can't help getting older, but you don't have to get old."

References

Chapter 1

Bortz, W. 1990. *We live too short and die too young.* New York: Bantam.

Costill, D. 1986. *Inside running, basics of sports physiology.* Dubuque, IA: Brown & Benchmark.

Fuch, T., et al. 1987. Cardiovascular changes for deterioration of aerobic capacity with aging in long distance runners. *Medicine and Science in Sport and Exercise* 19 (2): S61.

Heath, G. 1982. A physiological comparison of young and older endurance athletes. *Journal of Applied Physiology* 51 (3): 634-640.

Legwold, G. 1982. Masters competitors age little in ten years. *Physician and Sports Medicine* 10 (10): 27.

Levin, S. 1992. Can older be better? *Physician and Sports Medicine* 20 (7): 139-146.

McArdle, W., F. Katch, and V. Katch. 1996. *Exercise physiology.* Baltimore: Williams & Wilkins.

Pollock, M., et al. 1987. Effect of age and training on aerobic capacity and body composition of masters athletes. *Journal of Applied Physiology* 62 (2): 725-731.

Rogers, M., et al. 1990. Decline in $\dot{V}O_2$max with aging in master athletes and sedentary men. *Journal of Applied Physiology* 68 (5): 2195-2199.

Shafer, R., ed. 1996. *1996 rules of bicycle racing.* Colorado Springs: USA Cycling.

Spirudoso, W.W. 1995. *Physical dimensions of aging.* Champaign, IL: Human Kinetics.

Wilmore, J., and D. Costill. 1994. *Physiology of sport and exercise.* Champaign, IL: Human Kinetics.

Chapter 2

Anderson, O. 1995. How to tell when you're really fit. *Running Research News* 11 (1): 9.

Ericsson, K.A. 1990. Peak performance and age: An examination of peak performance in sports. In *Successful aging: Perspectives from the behavioral sciences,* edited by P.B. Baltes and M.M. Baltes. Cambridge, MA: Cambridge University Press.

Goldberg, R.J., et al. 1996. Factors associated with survival to 75 years of age in middle-aged men and women. *Archives of Internal Medicine* 156: 505-509.

Ryan, A. 1984. Sudden death: Running is not the culprit. *Physician and Sports Medicine* 12 (9): 29.

Shafer, R., ed. 1996. *1996 rules of bicycle racing.* Colorado Springs: USA Cycling.

Sherman, C. 1993. Sudden death during running: How great is the risk for middle-aged and older adults? *Physician and Sports Medicine* 21 (9): 93-99.

Stones, M.J., and A. Kozma. 1982. Cross-sectional, longitudinal, and secular age trends in athletic performances. *Experimental Aging Research* 8: 185-188.

VanCamp, S. 1984. The Fixx tragedy: A cardiologist's perspective. *Physician and Sports Medicine* 12 (9): 153-155.

Chapter 3

Bompa, T. 1994. *Theory and methodology of training.* Dubuque, IA: Kendall/Hunt.

Friel, J. 1996. *The cyclist's training bible.* Boulder, CO: VeloPress.

Janssen, P.G.J.M. 1987. *Training, lactate, pulse rate.* Oulu, Finland: Polar Electro Oy.

Kindermann, W., et al. 1979. The significance of the aerobic-anaerobic transition for the determination of work load intensities during endurance training. *European Journal of Applied Physiology* 42: 25-34.

Weltman, A. 1995. *The blood lactate response to exercise.* Champaign, IL: Human Kinetics.

Wenger, H.A., and G. Bell. 1986. The interactions of intensity, frequency, and duration of exercise training in altering cardiorespiratory fitness. *Sports Medicine* 3 (5): 346-356.

Chapter 4

Baker, A. 1995. Optimum crank arm length. *Performance Conditioning for Cycling* 2 (3): 7.

Friel, J. 1996. *The cyclist's training bible.* Boulder, CO: VeloPress.

Hickson, R.C., et al. 1985. Reduced training intensities and loss of aerobic power, endurance, and cardiac growth. *Journal of Applied Physiology* 58: 492-499.

Newsholme, E. 1988. Changes in plasma concentrations of aromatic and branched-chain amino acids during sustained exercise in man and their possible role in fatigue. *Acta Physiologica Scandinavica* 133: 115-121.

Scott, M., and J. Wappes. 1995. Use your head to choose a bike helmet. *Physician and Sports Medicine* 23 (8): 100w-100aa.

Wilmore, J., and D. Costill. 1994. *Physiology of sport and exercise.* Champaign, IL: Human Kinetics.

Chapter 5

Brogdowicz, G., and D. Lamb. 1986. Optimal use of fluids of varying formulations to minimize exercise-induced disturbances in homeostasis. *Sports Medicine* 3: 247-274.

Burke, E., ed. 1996. *High-tech cycling.* Champaign, IL: Human Kinetics.

Lovett, R. 1994. *The essential touring cyclist.* Camden, ME: Ragged Mountain Press.

Neufer, P.D., and D.L. Costill. 1986. Effects of exercise and carbohydrate composition on gastric emptying. *Medicine and Science in Sports and Exercise* 18: 658-662.

Chapter 6

Bompa, T. 1994. *Theory and methodology of training.* Dubuque, IA: Kendall/Hunt.

Friel, J. 1996. *The cyclist's training bible.* Boulder, CO: VeloPress.

Tracy, B. 1993. *Maximum achievement.* New York: Simon & Schuster.

Chapter 7

Anderson. O. 1992. Milk and sugar after workouts? They may be tickets to quicker recoveries. *Running Research News* 8 (6): 7-8.

Borer, K., D. Edington, and T. White, eds. 1983. *Frontiers of exercise biology.* Champaign, IL: Human Kinetics.

Cade, J., et al. 1991. Dietary intervention and training in swimmers. *European Journal of Applied Physiology* 63: 210-215.

Costill, D., et al. 1987. Effects of pre-exercise carbohydrate feedings on muscle glycogen use during exercise in well-trained runners. *European Journal of Applied Physiology* 56: 225-229.

Dodd, S., et al. 1984. Blood lactate disappearance at various intensities of recovery exercise. *Journal of Applied Physiology* 57: 1462-1465.

Dressendorfer, R., et al. 1985. Increased morning heart rate in runners: A valid sign of overtraining? *Physician and Sports Medicine* 13 (8): 77-86.

Francis, K., and T. Hoobler. 1987. Effects of aspirin on delayed muscle soreness. *Journal of Sports Medicine* 27: 333-337.

Ivy, J.L., et al. 1988. Muscle glycogen synthesis after exercise: Effect of time on carbohydrate ingestion. *Journal of Applied Physiology* 64: 1480-1485.

Newsholme, E., et al. 1988. Changes in plasma concentrations of aromatic and branched-chain amino acids during sustained exercise in man and their possible role in fatigue. *Acta Physiologica Scandinavica* 133: 115-121.

Newsholme, E., et al. 1989. Effects of sustained exercise on plasma amino acid concentrations on 5-hydroxyttryptamine metabolism in six different brain regions of the rat. *Acta Physiologica Scandinavica* 136: 473-481.

Parry-Billings, M., et al. 1992. Plasma amino acid concentrations in the overtraining syndrome: Possible effects on the immune system. *Medicine and Science in Sports and Exercise* 24: 1353-1358.

Ravussin, L., et al. 1979. Substrate utilization during prolonged exercise preceded by ingestion of 13C-glucose in glycogen depleted and control subjects. *Pflugers Archive* 382: 197-202.

Chapter 8

Anderson, B. 1980. *Stretching*. Bolinas, CA: Shelter.

Anderson, O. 1993. Should you run—or lift and run? *Running Research News* 9 (5): 9-10.

Anderson, O. 1995. What's the truth about running and bad knees? *Running Research News* 11 (8): 10-12.

Baker, A. 1995. *Bicycling medicine*. San Diego: Argo.

Bompa, T. 1993. *Periodization of strength*. Toronto, ON: Veritas.

Borms, J., et al. 1987. Optimal duration of static stretching exercises for improvements of coxo-femoral flexibility. *Journal of Sport Sciences* 5: 39-47.

Chapman, E.A., et al. 1972. Joint stiffness: Effects of exercise on young and old men. *Journal of Gerontology* 27: 218-221.

Felson, D.T., et al. 1988. Obesity and knee osteoarthritis. The Framingham study. *Annals of Internal Medicine* 109: 18-24.

Franks, B.D. 1983. Physical warm-up. In *Ergogenic aids in sport*, edited by M.H. Williams. Champaign, IL: Human Kinetics.

Friel, J. 1996. *The cyclist's training bible*. Boulder, CO: VeloPress.

Hatfield, F.C. 1982. *Flexibility training for sports*: PNF techniques.: Fitness Systems USA.

Holly, R.G., et al. 1980. Stretch-induced growth in chicken wing muscles: A new model of stretch hypertrophy. *American Journal of Physiology* 7: C62-C71.

Murray-Leslie, C.F., et al. 1977. The knees and ankles in sport and veteran military parachutists. *Annals of Rheumatic Diseases* 36: 327-331.

Noakes, T. 1991. *Lore of running*. Champaign, IL: Leisure Press.

Nordemar, R., et al. 1981. Physical training in rheumatoid arthritis: A controlled, long-term study. *Scandinavian Journal of Rheumatology* 10: 17-23.

Palmoski, M.J., et al. 1980. Joint motion in the absence of normal loading does not maintain normal articular cartilage. *Arthritis and Rheumatism* 23: 325-334.

Rovati, L.C. 1992. Clinical research in osteoarthritis: Design and results of short-term and long-term trials with disease-modifying drugs. *International Journal of Tissue Reactivity* 14 (5): 253-261.

Shellock, F.G., et al. 1985. Warming-up and stretching for improved physical performance and prevention of sports-related injuries. *Sports Medicine* 2: 267-278.

Spirduso, W.W. 1995. *Physical dimensions of aging.* Champaign, IL: Human Kinetics.

Vanderburgh, H., and S. Kaufman. 1983. Stretch and skeletal myotube growth: What is the physical to biochemical linkage? In *Frontiers of exercise biology,* edited by K. Borer, D. Edington, and T. White. Champaign, IL: Human Kinetics.

Wallin, D., et al. 1985. Improvement of muscle flexibility. A comparison of two techniques. *American Journal of Sports Medicine* 13: 263-268.

Chapter 9

Campbell, W.W., et al. 1994. Increased protein requirements in elderly people: New data and retrospective reassessments. *American Journal of Clinical Nutrition* 60 (4): 501-509.

Chen, I., et al. 1995. Why do low-fat, high-carbohydrate diets accentuate postprandial lipemia in patients with NIDDM? *Diabetes Care* 18 (1): 10-16.

Corti, M.C., et al. 1995. HDL cholesterol predicts coronary heart disease mortality in older persons. *Journal of the American Medical Association* 274: 539-544.

Devlin, J.T., et al. 1990. Amino acid metabolism after intense exercise. *American Journal of Physiology* 258: E249-E255.

Ekstedt, B., et al. Influence of dietary fat, cholesterol and energy on serum lipids at vigorous physical exertion. *Scandinavian Journal of Clinical Laboratory Investigation* 51: 437-442.

Evans, W.J., et al. 1983. Protein metabolism and endurance exercise. *Physician and Sports Medicine* 11: 63-72.

Foster-Powell, K., and J.B. Miller. 1995. International tables of glycemic index. *American Journal of Clinical Nutrition* 62: 871S-893S.

Friedman, J.E., and P. Lemon. 1989. Effect of chronic endurance exercise on the retention of dietary protein. *International Journal of Sports Medicine* 10: 118-123.

Holloszy, J.O. 1990. Utilization of fatty acids during exercise.

In *Biochemistry of exercise VII*, Vol. 21, edited by A.W. Taylor, P.D. Gollnick, and H.J. Green. Champaign, IL: Human Kinetics.

Jeppeson, Jorgen, et al. 1997. Effects of low-fat, high-carbohydrate diets on risk factors for ischemic heart disease in postmenopausal women. *American Journal of Clinical Nutrition* 65: 1027-1033.

Keys, A. 1980. *Seven countries: A multivariate analysis of death and coronary heart disease.* Cambridge, MA: Harvard University Press.

Kiens, B., et al. 1987. Lipoprotein lipase activity and intramuscular triglyceride stores after long-term, high-fat and high-carbohydrate diets in physically trained men. *Clinical Physiology* 7: 1-9.

Lambert, E.V., et al. 1994. Enhanced endurance in trained cyclists during moderate intensity exercise following two weeks adaptation to a high-fat diet. *European Journal of Applied Physiology and Occupational Physiology* 69 (4): 287-293.

Leddy, J., et al. 1997. Effect of a high- or low-fat diet on cardiovascular risk factors in male and female runners. *Medicine and Science in Sport and Exercise* 29 (1): 17-25.

Lemon, P. 1996. Is increased dietary protein necessary or beneficial for individuals with a physically active lifestyle? *Nutrition Reviews* 54: S169-S175.

Loosli, A.R. 1993. Reversing sports-related iron and zinc deficiencies. *Physician and Sports Medicine* 21 (6): 70-78.

McArdle, W., F. Katch, and V. Katch. 1996. *Exercise physiology.* Baltimore: Williams & Wilkins.

Meredith, C.N., et al. 1989. Dietary protein requirements and protein metabolism in endurance-trained men. *Journal of Applied Physiology* 66: 2850-2856.

Muoio, D.M., et al. 1994. Effect of dietary fat on metabolic adjustments to maximal $\dot{V}O_2$ and endurance in runners. *Medicine and Science in Sport and Exercise* 26: 81-88.

Personal communication with Dr. L. Cordain, Department of Exercise and Sport Science, Colorado State University, Fort Collins, Colorado 80523.

Spirduso, W.W. 1995. *Physical dimensions of aging.* Champaign, IL: Human Kinetics.

Thompson, P.D., et al. 1984. The effects of high-carbohydrate and high-fat diets on serum lipid and lipoprotein concentrations of endurance athletes. *Metabolism* 33: 1003-1010.

Wilmore, J., and D. Costill. 1994. *Physiology of sport and exercise.* Champaign, IL: Human Kinetics.

Chapter 10

Elliott, R. 1991. *The competitive edge.* Mountain View, CA: Tafnews Press.

Loehr, J. 1982. *Mental toughness training for sports.* New York: Penguin Books.

Loehr, J. 1994. *The new toughness training for sports.* New York: Penguin Books.

Lynch, J. 1987. *The total runner.* Toronto: Prentice Hall.

Lynch, J. 1992. *Thinking body, dancing mind.* New York: Bantam Books.

Orlick, T. 1980. *In pursuit of excellence.* Champaign, IL: Human Kinetics.

Tracy, B. 1993. *Maximum achievement.* New York: Fireside.

Ungerleider, S. 1996. *Mental training for peak performance.* Emmaus, PA: Rodale Press.

Wilcockson, J., ed. 1995. *Greg LeMond, the official story.* Boulder, CO: Inside Communications.

Chapter 11

Kienholz, M., and R. Pawlak. 1996. *Cycling in cyberspace.* San Francisco: Bicycle Books.

Oliver, P. 1995. *Bicycling, touring and mountain bike basics.* New York: Norton.

Perry, D. 1995. *Bike cult, the ultimate guide to human-powered vehicles.* New York: Four Walls Eight Windows.

Chapter 12

LeMond, G., and K. Gordis. 1988. *Greg LeMond's complete book of bicycling.* New York: Perigee.

Oliver, P. 1995. *Bicycling, touring and mountain bike basics.* New York: Norton.

Perry, D. 1995. *Bike cult.* New York: Four Walls Eight Windows.

Van der Plas, R. 1995. *The mountain bike book.* Mill Valley, CA: Bicycle Books.

Index

About the Author

Joe Friel has trained endurance athletes since 1980. His clients include elite amateur and professional road cyclists, mountain bikers, triathletes, and duathletes located around the world. He has a masters degree in exercise science, is an Elite-level USA Cycling coach, and serves on the USA Triathlon Coaching Certification Committee.

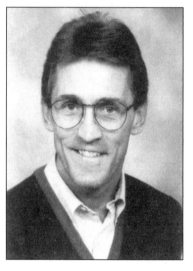

Joe is the author of *The CompuTrainer Workout Manual, The Cyclist's Training Bible,* and *The Triathlete's Training Bible.* He is a contributing editor to *Inside Triathlon* and *VeloNews* and frequently writes feature stories for *Performance Conditioning for Cycling.* He has written a weekly fitness column for the *Fort Collins Coloradoan* newspaper since 1981.

As an age-group competitor, Joe is a Colorado State Masters Triathlon champion, a Rocky Mountain region and Southwest region duathlon age-group champion, and is a perennial USA Triathlon All-American duathlete. A member of several national duathlon teams, Joe is a top five contender in world class events. In addition, he competes in road running and United States Cycling Federation races.

Joe speaks at workshops around the country on training and racing for endurance athletes and provides consulting services for corporations in the fitness industry. For information on coaching, speaking, or consulting services, contact him by e-mail at **jfriel@ultrafit.com** or fax him at 970-204-4221.

From his home at the foot of the Rocky Mountains in Fort Collins, Colorado, Joe enjoys mountain biking in the foothills with his wife Joyce, trail running with friends, and riding with his son Dirk, a professional bike racer.

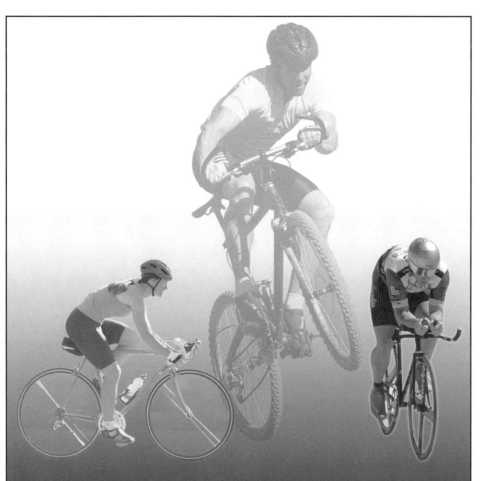